CUTANEOUS MELANOMA

CUTANEOUS MELANOMA
A POCKET GUIDE FOR DIAGNOSIS AND MANAGEMENT

Edited by

GIUSEPPE ARGENZIANO
University of Campania Luigi Vanvitelli, Naples, Italy

AIMILIOS LALLAS
Aristotle University of Thessaloniki, Thessaloniki, Greece

CATERINA LONGO
University of Modena and Reggio Emilia, Reggio Emilia, Italy

ELVIRA MOSCARELLA
University of Campania Luigi Vanvitelli, Naples;
Arcispedale S. Maria Nuova, IRCCS, Reggio Emilia, Italy

ATHANASSIOS KYRGIDIS
Aristotle University of Thessaloniki, Thessaloniki, Greece

GERARDO FERRARA
Macerata General Hospital, Macerata, Italy

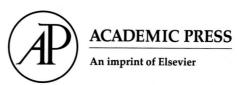

ACADEMIC PRESS
An imprint of Elsevier

Academic Press is an imprint of Elsevier
125 London Wall, London EC2Y 5AS, United Kingdom
525 B Street, Suite 1800, San Diego, CA 92101-4495, United States
50 Hampshire Street, 5th Floor, Cambridge, MA 02139, United States
The Boulevard, Langford Lane, Kidlington, Oxford OX5 1GB, United Kingdom

Notices
Knowledge and best practice in this field are constantly changing. As new research and experience broaden our understanding, changes in research methods, professional practices, or medical treatment may become necessary.

Practitioners and researchers must always rely on their own experience and knowledge in evaluating and using any information, methods, compounds, or experiments described herein. In using such information or methods they should be mindful of their own safety and the safety of others, including parties for whom they have a professional responsibility.

To the fullest extent of the law, neither the Publisher nor the authors, contributors, or editors, assume any liability for any injury and/or damage to persons or property as a matter of products liability, negligence or otherwise, or from any use or operation of any methods, products, instructions, or ideas contained in the material herein.

Library of Congress Cataloging-in-Publication Data
A catalog record for this book is available from the Library of Congress

British Library Cataloguing-in-Publication Data
A catalogue record for this book is available from the British Library

ISBN: 978-0-12-804000-3

For information on all Academic Press publications visit our website at
https://www.elsevier.com/books-and-journals

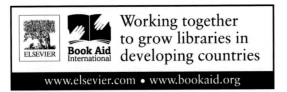

Working together
to grow libraries in
developing countries

www.elsevier.com • www.bookaid.org

Publisher: Mica Haley
Acquisition Editor: Rafael Teixeira
Editorial Project Manager: Tracy Tufaga
Production Project Manager: Chris Wortley
Designer: Mark Rogers

Typeset by Thomson Digital

Contents

Contributors

Antoni Bennassar   University of Barcelona, Barcelona; Research Center of the Biomedical Network of Rare Diseases (CIBERER), Carlos III Health Institute, Madrid, Spain

Stefania Borsari   Arcispedale Santa Maria Nuova—IRCCS, Reggio Emilia, Italy

Gabriella Brancaccio   University of Campania Luigi Vanvitelli, Naples, Italy

Stephane Dalle   Lyon 1 University, Cancer Research Center of Lyon, Lyon, France

Maria Concetta Fargnoli   University of L'Aquila, L'Aquila, Italy

Paolo Fava   University of Turin, Turin, Italy

Gerardo Ferrara   Macerata General Hospital, Macerata, Italy

Maria T. Fierro   University of Turin, Turin, Italy

Gianfrancesco Gallino   IRCCS Foundation of the National Cancer Institute, Milan, Italy

Athanassios Kyrgidis   Aristotle University of Thessaloniki, Thessaloniki, Greece

Aimilios Lallas   Aristotle University of Thessaloniki, Thessaloniki, Greece

Caterina Longo   University of Modena and Reggio Emilia, Reggio Emilia, Italy

Josep Malvehy   University of Barcelona, Barcelona; Research Center of the Biomedical Network of Rare Diseases (CIBERER), Carlos III Health Institute, Madrid, Spain

Ilaria Mattavelli   IRCCS Foundation of the National Cancer Institute, Milan, Italy

Andrea Maurichi   IRCCS Foundation of the National Cancer Institute, Milan, Italy

Elvira Moscarella   University of Campania Luigi Vanvitelli, Naples; Arcispedale S. Maria Nuova, IRCCS, Reggio Emilia, Italy

Roberto Patuzzo   IRCCS Foundation of the National Cancer Institute, Milan, Italy

Cristina Pellegrini   University of L'Aquila, L'Aquila, Italy

Ketty Peris   Institute of Dermatology, Catholic University of the Sacred Heart, Rome, Italy

Susana Puig   University of Barcelona, Barcelona; Research Center of the Biomedical Network of Rare Diseases (CIBERER), Carlos III Health Institute, Madrid, Spain

Pietro Quaglino   University of Turin, Turin, Italy

Mario Santinami   IRCCS Foundation of the National Cancer Institute, Milan, Italy

Luc Thomas   Lyon 1 University, Cancer Research Center of Lyon, Lyon, France

Sergi Vidal-Sicart   University of Barcelona, Barcelona; Research Center of the Biomedical Network of Rare Diseases (CIBERER), Carlos III Health Institute, Madrid, Spain

Cutaneous Melanoma: A Pocket Guide for Diagnosis and Management

First and foremost, it is my honor and my pleasure indeed to write a few lines on this "short and sweet," albeit comprehensive and substantive, pocket guide for diagnosis and management of cutaneous melanoma. In the past decade so much exciting has happened and is going to happen on the subject matter of melanoma, particularly relevant for all affected with melanoma and its uncertain history. No doubt, the preposterous increase in data and information about cutaneous melanoma challenges dermatologists, medical and surgical oncologists, as well as all doctors involved with the diagnosis and management of patients with cutaneous melanoma.

Geppi (Giuseppe) Argenziano and his colleagues deserve to be applauded for undertaking the effort to summarize the "status quo" of cutaneous melanoma in 2017. On a personal note, it is an enjoyment to see that, my friend and colleague for two decades, Geppi has returned to Naples, this vibrant and unique Italian city, and will lead the great tradition of dermatology at the Second University of Naples with energy, dedication, and vision with a new and specific focus on the secondary prevention (early detection) of melanoma. This pocket guide, however, encompasses the whole spectrum of prevention of cutaneous melanoma from primary to tertiary prevention, the latter better known as treatment. Geppi and a team of committed and dedicated experts contributing to this melanoma guide are well aware of its transitory aspect due to the rapid development of research in melanoma and the fast-changing landscape of health service provision in this field. The content of this book spans from epidemiology and risk factors, all the up-to-date facets of clinical diagnosis, to a stage-appropriate approach of treatment. The seventh and final chapter addresses special clinical situations with familial melanoma and multiple primary melanoma as well as pediatric melanoma and atypical Spitz tumor mentioning but two of the most relevant examples for patients/consumers and doctors alike. Each chapter is prepared in a systematic and concise way and given the distinctiveness of the chapters/subchapters is following an individual ductus including introduction, discussion, and at the end of each chapter/subchapter a compilation of references, making this pocket guide a complete reading experience.

May this pocket guide for the diagnosis and management of cutaneous melanoma be of help, direction, and guidance for all those interested and keen to read and learn about the "state-of-the-art" knowledge of this most mysterious and secretive cancer lying before our eyes.

H. Peter Soyer, MD, FACD, FAHMS

Professor and Chair in Dermatology,
Dermatology Research Centre,
The University of Queensland,
Diamantina Institute, Brisbane, Australia

Melanoma Epidemiology

Athanassios Kyrgidis

Aristotle University of Thessaloniki, Thessaloniki, Greece

1 INCIDENCE AND MORTALITY

The incidence of melanoma is rising faster than that of any other type of cancer while mortality rates are not rising or remain stable in many countries [1–7]:

- US incidence of melanoma: 60,000 new cases per year (about 4% of all newly diagnosed cancers).
- US average mortality: 8000 people per year.
- Approximately 1 out of 50–60 Americans alive today will develop melanoma in their lifetime (Lifetime Risk of Developing Cancer: 2.1%, approximately).
- Based on 2008–12 cases in the United States, the age-adjusted number of new cases of melanoma of the skin is 21.6 per 100,000 men and women per year. The age-adjusted number of deaths is 2.7 per 100,000 men and women per year [1,8].

Cutaneous Melanoma. http://dx.doi.org/10.1016/B978-0-12-804000-3.00001-6

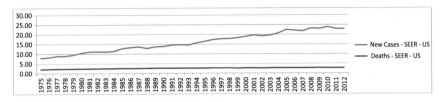

FIGURE 1.1 **Trends in melanoma: new cases and deaths per 100,000 persons in the United States in the past 30 years [8].**

In the United States, incidence rates for new melanoma of the skin have been rising on average 1.4% each year over the past 10 years. Death rates have been stable over 2002–12. There are two possible explanations:

- Patients present at an earlier stage of tumor development.
- There has been a significant increase in screening for melanoma with a large number of very borderline and very thin melanomas diagnosed.

Fig. 1.1, which presents mortality and death trends in the United States in the past 30 years, clearly demonstrates this fact.

2 SURVIVAL

Based on data from SEER 18, 2005–11, the relative 5-year melanoma-specific survival (survival in the absence of other causes of death, which is calculated using survival life tables) was 91.5%, meaning that fewer than 9 out of 100 patients diagnosed with melanoma will die of the disease in the next 5 years from diagnosis.

Figs. 1.2 and 1.3 present, respectively, frequency and impact in 5-year relative survival of each melanoma stage when diagnosed:

- Localized: cancer cells are confined to the primary site
- Regional: cancer cells have spread to the regional lymph nodes

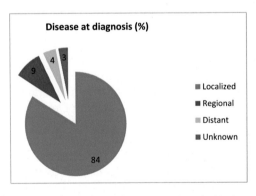

FIGURE 1.2 **Melanoma stage at diagnosis.** *Source: Adapted with changes from SEER cancer statistics factsheets: melanoma of the skin. Bethesda, MD: National Cancer Institute.*

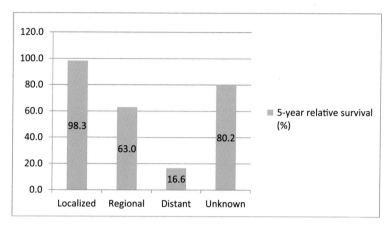

FIGURE 1.3 **Five-year relative survival dependent on stage at diagnosis.** *Source: Adapted with changes from SEER cancer statistics factsheets: melanoma of the skin. Bethesda, MD: National Cancer Institute.*

TABLE 1.1 Five-Year Relative (Disease-Specific) Survival of Patients Diagnosed With Melanoma in the United States in the Past 30 Years

	Year							
	1975	1980	1985	1990	1995	1999	2003	2007
5-Year relative survival (%)	81.8	83.9	86.1	89.2	90.1	92.3	93.2	93.2

- Distant: cancer cells have metastasized
- Unknown: for those patients who were not staged on diagnosis

The trends in relative survival have been rising, from a relative survival of 81.8% back in 1975 to a relative survival of 93.2% in 2007 (Table 1.1). In Australia between 1982–86 and 2007–11, 5-year relative survival from melanoma skin cancer improved from 85 to 90% [9].

3 EUROPE

In Europe, cutaneous melanoma represents 1–2% of all malignant tumors:

- Incidence of melanoma: 18,000 new cases per year
- Average mortality: 5000 people per year [1,7]

One-year, 3-year, and 5-year prevalence of melanoma is 87,285, 247,837, and 391,316 persons, respectively, in Europe (Fig. 1.4). In the European Union (27 states), the same 1-year, 3-year, and 5-year numbers are 71,476, 204,015, and 323,467 persons, respectively [10].

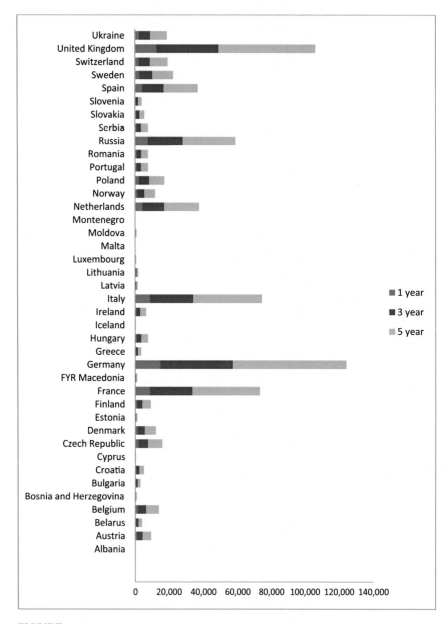

FIGURE 1.4 **One-year, 3-year, and 5-year prevalence of melanoma in 39 European countries.** *Source: Data from EUCAN cancer factsheets. Lyon, France: Cancéropôle Lyon, Auvergne, Rhone-Alps (CLARA).*

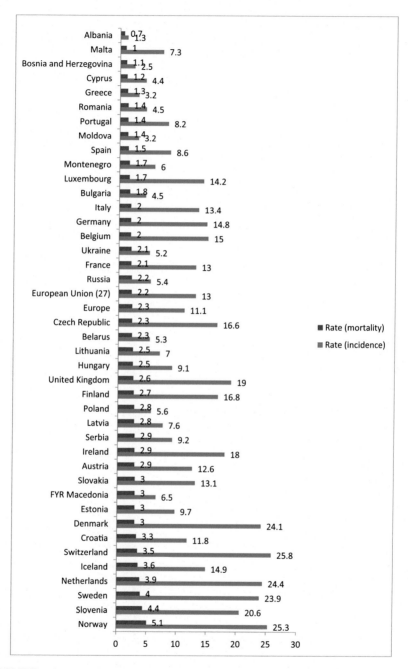

FIGURE 1.5 **Incidence and mortality rates of melanoma in 42 European countries (per 100,000 inhabitants).** *Source: Data from EUCAN cancer factsheets. Lyon, France: Cancéropôle Lyon, Auvergne, Rhone-Alps (CLARA).*

In Europe, incidence and mortality rates for melanoma are reported to be different among various countries, with Norway and Sweden being those with the higher incidence rates (Fig. 1.5) [10].

In Fig. 1.5, very pronounced differences in both incidence and mortality among different European countries can be noted:

- The incidence of melanoma shows a characteristic geographical variability.
- Individuals with Celtic ancestry appear to have the highest predisposition to develop this type of cancer [1].
- As Celtic people migrate to more temperate regions, the incidence of melanoma increases: this is particularly evident in *Australia*, where melanoma is expected to account for 10.2% of all new cancers diagnosed in 2015 [9].
- Of note, in Australia, the age-standardized incidence rate increased from 27 cases per 100,000 persons in 1982 to 48 per 100,000 persons in 2011 probably due to a very aggressive screening policy for melanoma [7].

4 RACE/ETHNICITY

Melanoma is rare in nonwhites (Caucasians: Asian/black populations = 20:1) and—when present—it is mostly confined to nonpigmented sites (subungual regions, palms, and soles) [11]. Despite a lower incidence, mortality rate is higher [8].

- Fig. 1.6 presents the US standardized incidence ratios for melanoma of the skin for ethnicity and sex (number of new cases per 100,000 persons adjusted for race/ethnicity and sex) [8].

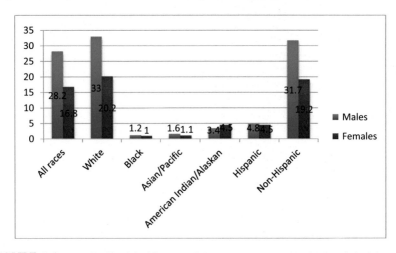

FIGURE 1.6 **Standardized incidence ratios per 100,000 persons by race/ethnicity and sex: for melanoma of the skin [8].**

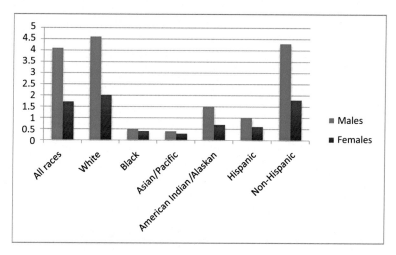

FIGURE 1.7 **Standardized mortality ratios per 100,000 persons by race/ethnicity and sex: for melanoma of the skin [8].**

- Fig. 1.7 presents the US standardized mortality ratios for melanoma of the skin for ethnicity and sex (number of deaths per 100,000 persons adjusted for race/ethnicity and sex) [8].

5 AGE

Melanoma is extremely rare prior to puberty.

- The incidence increases with age until the fifth decade. The median age at diagnosis is 63 years [8,12], which is a relatively young age for a cancer patient (Fig. 1.8).

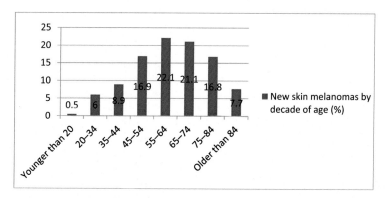

FIGURE 1.8 **Decade of age of patients diagnosed with melanoma. SEER 2008–12, all races, both sexes [8].**

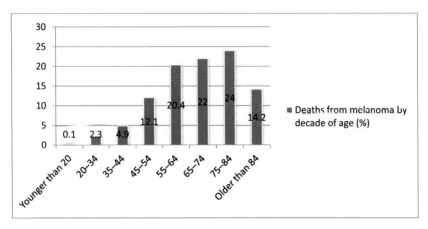

FIGURE 1.9 **Decade of age of patients dying from melanoma. SEER 2008–12, all races, both sexes [8].**

- Death rates are higher among the middle-aged and elderly [12]. The number of deaths was 2.7 per 100,000 men and women per year based on 2008–12 deaths. Deaths by decade of age are presented in Fig. 1.9.

6 BODY LOCATION

The distribution of skin melanoma in the different body areas is not homogeneous. Using the first invasive cutaneous melanoma as reference lesion, Lachiewicz et al. reported the body site distribution among non-Hispanic white adults collected by the SEER 17 Registry Program from 2000 to 2004:

- 43% on the extremities
- 34% on the trunk
- 12% on the face/ears
- 7% on the scalp/neck
- 4% at other/unclassified sites [13]

References

[1] Bataille V, de Vries E. Melanoma—part 1: epidemiology, risk factors, and prevention. BMJ 2008;337:a2249.
[2] Demierre MF. Epidemiology and prevention of cutaneous melanoma. Curr Treat Options Oncol 2006;7(3):181–6.
[3] Jemal A, Siegel R, Ward E, Murray T, Xu J, Smigal C, et al. Cancer statistics, 2006. CA Cancer J Clin 2006;56(2):106–30.
[4] Kyrgidis A, Tzellos T, Mocellin S, Apalla Z, Lallas A, Pilati P, et al. Sentinel lymph node biopsy followed by lymph node dissection for localised primary cutaneous melanoma. Cochrane Database Syst Rev 2015;5:CD010307.

[5] Markovic SN, Erickson LA, Rao RD, Weenig RH, Pockaj BA, Bardia A, et al. Malignant melanoma in the 21st century, part 1: epidemiology, risk factors, screening, prevention, and diagnosis. Mayo Clin Proc 2007;82(3):364–80.

[6] Thompson JF, Scolyer RA, Kefford RF. Cutaneous melanoma. Lancet 2005;365(9460): 687–701.

[7] Forsea AM, del Marmol V, de Vries E, Bailey EE, Geller AC. Melanoma incidence and mortality in Europe: new estimates, persistent disparities. Br J Dermatol 2012;167(5):1124–30.

[8] SEER cancer statistics factsheets: melanoma of the skin. Bethesda, MD: National Cancer Institute.

[9] Melanoma skin cancer in Australia. Australian Government Cancer Australia. Available from: https://melanoma.canceraustralia.gov.au/statistics.

[10] EUCAN cancer factsheets. Lyon, France: Cancéropôle Lyon, Auvergne, Rhone-Alps (CLARA).

[11] Goldenberg A, Vujic I, Sanlorenzo M, Ortiz-Urda S. Melanoma risk perception and prevention behavior among African-Americans: the minority melanoma paradox. Clin Cosmet Investig Dermatol 2015;8:423–9.

[12] Tsai S, Balch C, Lange J. Epidemiology and treatment of melanoma in elderly patients. Nat Rev Clin Oncol 2010;7(3):148–52.

[13] Lachiewicz AM, Berwick M, Wiggins CL, Thomas NE. Epidemiologic support for melanoma heterogeneity using the Surveillance, Epidemiology, and End Results Program. J Invest Dermatol 2008;128(5):1340–2.

Further Reading

Guy GP Jr, Thomas CC, Thompson T, Watson M, Massetti GM, Richardson LC. Vital signs: melanoma incidence and mortality trends and projections—United States, 1982–2030. MMWR Morb Mortal Wkly Rep 2015;64(21):591–6.

Khosrotehrani K, Dasgupta P, Byrom L, Youlden DR, Baade PD, Green AC. Melanoma survival is superior in females across all tumour stages but is influenced by age. Arch Dermatol Res 2015;307(8):731–40.

CHAPTER

2

Risk Factors

Athanassios Kyrgidis

Aristotle University of Thessaloniki, Thessaloniki, Greece

Cutaneous Melanoma. http://dx.doi.org/10.1016/B978-0-12-804000-3.00002-8

1 SEX

Melanoma is not more common in any sex, as the total incidence rate in Europe is 11.4 patients/100,000 men and 11.0 patients/100,000 women. It can be argued that as far as Europe is concerned, only a very slight male preponderance exists.

On the contrary, the mortality rates are evidently higher for men (2.8/100,000) as compared to those for women (1.8/100,000) even adjusting for tumor thickness. It has therefore been suggested that there could be some—yet—unknown sex-related factors that may improve survival in females.

2 RACE

Melanoma can be considered a disease of the white race, as the proportion of the risk of developing melanoma between Caucasians and Asian/ black populations is approximately 20:1.

In nonwhites melanoma is rare and mostly confined to nonpigmented sites such as the subungual regions, the palms of the hand, and the soles of the feet. This preference of melanoma in white people is for the most part attributable to non-Hispanic whites, which is a subgroup of white people (Fig. 2.1). In nonwhite patients, although the incidence is lower, the mortality rate is higher; this has been argued to be attributable to late diagnosis.

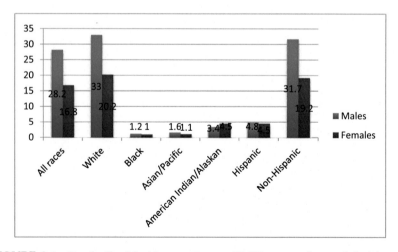

FIGURE 2.1 **Standardized incidence ratios per 100,000 persons by race/ethnicity and sex: for melanoma of the skin [1].**

Moreover, the incidence of melanoma shows a characteristic geographical variability. Individuals with Celtic ancestry appear to have the highest risk for developing melanoma. It has been suggested that as people of Celtic ancestry migrate to more temperate regions, the incidence of melanoma increases: this is particularly evident in Australia, where melanoma is expected to account for 10.2% of all new cancers diagnosed in 2015. Of note, in Australia, the age-standardized incidence rate increased from 27 cases per 100,000 persons in 1982 to 48 per 100,000 persons in 2011.

3 AGE

Melanoma often afflicts young, productive members of the society, with one-fourth of melanoma cases diagnosed in the United States occurring in individuals before the age of 40.

Melanomas diagnosed in those below 40 years of age are more likely to be thinner tumors with a better prognosis. Expectedly, there is an increase of melanoma with age like all other cancers.

Although all ages are at risk, melanoma is extremely rare prior to puberty; thereafter the incidence increases with age; the median age at diagnosis ranges from 45 to 55 years depending on the population studied.

4 SOMATOMETRIC CONDITIONS

Melanoma risk has been reported to be 17% higher per each 5-cm height increment in females and 13% higher per each 5-cm height increment in males, as shown in a pooled analysis of Nordic data.

Melanoma risk was reported to be 31% higher in overweight [body mass index (BMI) 25–29.9] and obese (BMI >30) men, compared with that in men whose BMI was lower than 25. Melanoma risk may not be associated with BMI in women; however, this may reflect mutual confounding between body size and sun exposure (e.g., larger women could self-limit their public sun exposure).

5 SUN EXPOSURE (INTERMITTENT OR CHRONIC)

The risk of melanoma has been reported to increase with intermittent intense sun exposure to high-intensity sunlight (e.g., sunbathing or holidaying in a place with strong sunlight), than to chronic sunlight exposure (e.g., being in an outdoor occupation).

Melanoma risk is 60% higher in people with the highest level of intermittent sun exposure when compared with those with the lowest, but this effect was limited to populations outside the United Kingdom, the United States, Canada, or Australia.

However, the true relationship between melanoma and sun exposure is very difficult to clearly describe because of other innate risk factors such as skin and hair color that confound this relationship.

On the contrary, chronic sun exposure—for which a well-established relationship with the risk of epithelial (nonmelanoma) skin cancer exists—has not been reported to also increase melanoma risk. In fact, it might even protect from developing melanoma.

With regard to the occupational sun exposure, it is still reported that it may increase the risk for developing melanoma when compared to no sun exposure at all.

Animal studies and population-based studies point to the ultraviolet (UVB) radiation emitted by the sun as a major exogenous causative factor; again whether UVB is more harmful than UVA is still not really established. A study conducted in the United States that did not separate UVA from UVB reported that adolescent and young adult melanoma risk, and possibly also childhood melanoma risk, were higher in geographical areas with higher ultraviolet levels.

The data mentioned previously are in contrast with the case in nonmelanoma skin cancer (NMSC). More specifically, basal cell carcinoma (BCC) risk is 43% higher in people who work outdoors, compared with in those who do not. Squamous cell carcinoma (SCC) risk is 77% higher in outdoor workers compared with that in indoor workers. Both these associations are stronger in countries nearer the equator. Unlike NMSC, melanoma does not show a preference for skin parts exposed to sunlight. The latter fact makes the correlation between UV exposure and the incidence melanoma more trivial. To further complicate this matter, despite the fact that melanin is widely thought to protect human skin against the mutagenic effects of UV radiation, the development of melanoma among albinos is very rare. The latter fact, furthermore, questions the role of UV light in melanoma genesis.

5.1 Artificial UV Sources

Use of UV-emitting tanning devices (mostly tanning beds) is considered as a cause of melanoma, and as a probable cause of SCC, based on limited evidence. Still there is no general consensus that artificial UV is harmful and the plausible positive relationship is associated with a small relative risks. More specifically, melanoma risk has been found to be 16%–25% higher in people who have ever used a tanning bed at any age, when compared to those who never used a tanning bed, although risk may vary by region. Melanoma risk was reported to be up to 59% higher in people who first used a tanning bed before the age of 35, when compared to those who never used a tanning bed.

Of note, SCC risk has been reported to be at least 67% higher in people who have ever used a tanning bed at any age, when compared to in those who never used a tanning bed. BCC risk has been reported to be up to 29% higher in people who have ever used a tanning bed (at any age), when compared to those who never used a tanning bed. It was reported to be 40% higher in people who first used a tanning bed before age 25. Few case–control studies concluded that melanoma and BCC risk were increased in people who have ever used a tanning bed, irrespective of the number of tanning bed–related burns. A cohort study also concluded that early onset melanoma and BCC risk may increase by tanning bed use. White young females are the commonest users of tanning beds. Because higher melanoma incidence rates have been noted in this subgroup of people, those incidence rates have been attributed to the higher tanning bed use rates.

Tanning bed use could be even more harmful for specific groups of patients: children; people with skin phototypes I or II, many moles (nevi) and/or history of frequent childhood sunburn, and/or sun-damaged skin; and people wearing cosmetics or taking medications that may enhance their UV sensitivity.

5.2 Sunburns

Melanoma risk is more than doubled in people with a history of sunburn (often caused by intermittent exposure to high-intensity sunlight), compared with people who have never been sunburned, as two meta-analyses have shown. A pooled analysis found that the risk for melanoma increases by 2–3 times in women who had over 26 "painful" or "severe" sunburns in their lifetime. This increased risk of melanoma is irrelevant of whether sunburn occurred in childhood or adulthood.

5.3 Sunscreens

Regarding the possible protective effect of sunscreen use to minimize the risk of melanoma, the results of epidemiological studies do not support such a protective effect of sunscreen use so far. Of note, because of the long lag time for melanoma development and because of the probably small magnitude of the relative risk ratios associated with the plausible—protective—sunscreen use, it may take a long time to accurately assess this relationship. The impact of sunscreen use on skin cancer risk will likely remain unclear, due largely to methodological limitations and other behaviors that may accompany (and confound) sunscreen use.

This apparently conflicting evidence could be owing to the multifactorial model of melanoma carcinogenesis with complex interactions between genotype, phenotype, and environment [2].

6 MOLES/NEVI

Clark (dysplastic) nevi are histopathologically defined by the presence of an architectural disorder with some fusion of rete ridges, lymphocytic infiltrate in the upper dermis, and nuclear atypia of the melanocytes in the nest. Clark nevi are often defined clinically (also clinically defined as atypical nevi) and usually have a diameter not less than 5 mm with a hazy border and with irregular pigmentation. People with atypical nevi have a 4–10 times higher risk for melanoma when compared to those people who do not have atypical nevi. Of note, melanoma, if it will arise, may appear on prior normal skin and not necessarily near the atypical lesion. Therefore, atypical nevi are considered markers that allow the identification of people at an increased risk for melanoma. Nevi do appear with age with a steady increase in childhood and early adulthood and thereafter there is a steady decline from middle age onwards. Most nevi are genetically determined. Sun exposure can increase the number of nevi, with chronic sun exposure being more influential than the number of sunburns in the past. The senescence of nevi along with increasing age could be related to genes like the p16 that might have a role in the disappearance of nevi with age. The total nevi number has also been reported to correlate with telomere length with higher number of nevi in those subjects with longer telomers; it has even been proposed that nevi could be useful as a marker of aging.

Nevi number is a very useful predictor for melanoma; it is considered the most commonly associated risk factor for melanoma and it can easily be documented in all Caucasian populations. People with a large number (over 100) of common moles exhibit a melanoma risk that is nearly 7 times higher than those people with very few (less than 15) moles. Melanoma risk increases by around 2% for every additional common mole, as Olsen et al. reported.

7 PHOTOTYPE

People with fair complexion, blue gray or green eyes, red or blond hair, and lots of freckles are at higher risk of developing melanoma as compared to people with other skin types. Of those fair skin-colored people, those with red and blond hair have an approximately two-fold higher risk for melanoma development when compared to those with dark hair. Because a similar risk pattern of sensitivity to sunlight exists, clinicians and investigators have devised a phototype classification that takes into account these features, as shown in Table 2.1. Using this classification as reference it has been suggested—based on available evidence—that melanoma risk is more than doubled in people with skin phototype I compared

TABLE 2.1   Skin Phototype Classification

Phototype	Constitutive skin color	Sunburn and tanning	Immediate tanning	Delayed tanning
I	Ivory white	Burns easily, never tans	−	−
II	White	Burns easily, tans minimally	±	±
III	White	Burns and tans moderately	+	+
IV	Beige-olive, lightly tanned	Burns minimally, tans moderately	++	++
V	Moderate brown or tanned	Rarely burns, tans profusely	+++	+++
VI	Dark brown or black	Never burns, tans profusely	+++	+++

with people with skin phototype IV. A recent metaanalysis reported that melanoma risk is almost double for all people with skin phototype II, and is 35% higher for people with skin phototype III, always compared with the melanoma risk for those people having skin phototype IV.

7.1 Eye Color

The same metaanalysis by Olsen et al. concluded that the risk for melanoma is 57% higher in people with blue/blue-gray eyes, as compared with that in dark-eyed people. People with green/gray/hazel eyes have a 51% greater melanoma risk again compared with dark-eyed people. Notably, BCC and SCC risk has been reported to also be more prevalent in people with blue/green-blue/green-gray eyes, when compared with that in dark-eyed people.

7.2 Hair Color

Melanoma risk has been reported to be triple in people with red/red-blonde hair, as compared to that in dark-haired people. It has been reported to be double in blonde people, and 46% higher in people with light brown hair, as compared with that in dark-haired people. This trend is similar in NMSC.

7.3 Freckles

People with freckles have a double risk for melanoma, when compared with people without freckles, according to Olsen et al. This effect of freckles has been reported to be independent of the number of moles in those people with freckles.

8 PERSONAL OR FAMILY HISTORY OF MELANOMA

Patients with melanoma have an increased risk of developing a second melanoma. The incidence of multiple primary melanomas ranges from 1.3% to 8.0% in large retrospective series. People with first-degree relatives affected with melanoma are at higher risk for melanoma. The risk for melanoma almost doubles in people with a family history of the same disease, versus in people without any such family history. Fallah et al. in their Nordic Registries Cohort study reported that this risk is higher if the affected relative has been aged under 30 at diagnosis, or if more than one first-degree relatives were affected. To summarize, it has been suggested that around 10% of all melanoma cases can be attributed to inherited risk.

9 GENETIC CONDITIONS

Melanoma risk is higher in Europeans with CDKN2A mutation, characteristic of familial atypical multiple mole melanoma (FAMMM); around 6 out of 10 carriers of the mutation develop melanoma by the age 80.

9.1 Li–Fraumeni Syndrome

Melanoma and NMSC risk may be increased in Li–Fraumeni syndrome (LFS): TP53 encodes p53, the so-called "genome guardian" because of its pivotal role in cell cycle arrest following DNA damage, which preserves cells from propagating errors in the genetic code. Somatic mutations of this gene exist in about 50% of all sporadic tumors. Germline mutations of TP53 can be found in the LFS, a cancer syndrome characterized by the predisposition to a wide range of tumors. The classical LFS requisites the following criteria: (1) sarcoma diagnosed before 45 years; (2) a first-degree relative aged under 45 years with any type of malignancy; (3) another first- or second-degree relative in the same familial line with any cancer aged under 45 years or a sarcoma at any age. Mutations in TP53 are found in 77% of classical LFS families. Many studies have indicated an association with a wider range of tumors, including melanoma, but since the absolute number of melanoma cases is low, there is some debate regarding whether this tumor type is truly a rare manifestation of LFS. There is also some evidence that subjects belonging to other family cancer syndromes with an excess of all cancers in general may be more prone to melanoma and this is particularly relevant for families with pancreas, brain, and breast cancers. Other family cancer syndromes such as neurofibromatosis have also been associated with a higher prevalence of melanoma.

9.2 Xeroderma Pigmentosum

Xeroderma pigmentosum (XP) is a rare genetic disease inherited in an autosomal recessive manner (its estimated prevalence is 1:1,000,000 in the United States and 1:100,000 in Japan). It is characterized by sun sensitivity, ocular damage, and a 1000-fold increased risk of cutaneous (BCC, squamous carcinoma, as well as melanoma) and ocular neoplasms. XP is known to be associated with mutations in the following genes: XPA, ERCC3 (XPB), XPC, ERCC2 (XPD), DDB2 (XPE), ERCC4 (XPF), ERCC5 (XPG), and POLH (XP-V). Mutations in XPA and XPC account for about 50% of XP cases. These genetic alterations are responsible for impaired nucleotide excision repair, which ultimately leads to genomic instability and carcinogenic mutations following DNA damage by ultraviolet radiation. Currently no cure exists for XP. The DNA damage is cumulative and irreversible. Management is limited to avoidance of exposure to damaging ultraviolet light by staying indoors with sunlight blocked out, and by means of protective clothing, sunscreens, and sunglasses.

9.3 Hereditary Retinoblastoma

The RB1 gene was the first tumor suppressor gene that had been cloned. The classical two-hit hypothesis is based on the observation that individuals carrying RB1 germline mutations develop retinoblastoma when the remaining wild-type copy is lost somatically. The penetrance of this cancer susceptibility gene germline mutations is approximately 90%, and tumors are generally bilateral. Hereditary retinoblastoma occurs in the early childhood and the 5-year survival rate is about 90% if the tumor is diagnosed when still confined to the eye. The activity of the retinoblastoma protein (pRb)—a well-characterized cell cycle inhibitor—is regulated by p16INK4A through its negative effect on the activity of the cyclin D-CDK4/CDK6 complexes, which phosphorylates and thereby inactivates the transcriptional suppressor function of pRb. An excess risk of cancers other than retinoblastoma has been reported in RB1 germline mutation carriers, with a cumulative incidence of adult cancer of approximately 70%. Besides an increased risk of epithelial cancers in older adults, this figure is largely due to the early onset sarcomas and melanoma: in particular, melanoma accounts for about 7%–8% of nonretinoblastoma malignancies in this cancer-prone population.

10 IMMUNE SUPPRESSION

Melanoma risk is 2.4 times higher in organ transplant recipients compared with that in the general population. Melanoma risk is 80% higher in people with Crohn's disease. Melanoma risk is 23% higher in people with ulcerative colitis. Melanoma risk among people with inflammatory bowel disease (IBD; including Crohn's disease and ulcerative colitis) is not associated with treatment type received for the disease.

A cohort study reported that melanoma risk can be up to 11 times higher in people with severe psoriasis. Melanoma risk is 50% higher in people with HIV or AIDS.

10.1 Previous Irradiation

Radiotherapy for a previous cancer increases the risk for melanoma. It is estimated to have caused 17.9% of second primary melanoma cases in women and 2.8% of second primary melanoma cases in men in 2010. A cohort study reported that melanoma but also NMSC risk is 14% higher in people who receive at least one computed tomography (CT) scan of the

TABLE 2.2   Risk Factors for Melanoma

Risk factor	Action	References	Quality of the evidence
Male sex	Increases mortality, not incidence	[3–6]	Convincing evidence
Height	Increases with height	[7]	Probable evidence
BMI	Increases with weight	[8]	Probable evidence
Intermittent sun exposure	Increases incidence	[9–11]	Convincing evidence
Chronic sun exposure	Does not increase incidence	[9–13]	Probable evidence
UVA, UVB	Increases childhood, adolescent, and young adult melanoma risk	[14]	Probable evidence
Tanning beds	Increases incidence	[15,16]	Probable evidence
Episodes of sunburns	Increase incidence	[9–11,17]	Convincing evidence
Use of sunscreens	Decreases incidence	[15,18–23]	Probable evidence
Moles/nevi	Increase incidence	[9–11,24,25]	Convincing evidence
Lighter skin phototypes	Increase incidence	[24,25]	Convincing evidence
Lighter eye color	Increases incidence	[24,25]	Probable evidence

TABLE 2.2   Risk Factors for Melanoma (*cont.*)

Risk factor	Action	References	Quality of the evidence
Lighter hair color	Increases incidence	[24,25]	Probable evidence
Freckles	Increase incidence	[24,25]	Convincing evidence
Personal or familial history of melanoma	Increases incidence	[9–11,24–26]	Convincing evidence
Genetic conditions: Li–Fraumeni syndrome; xeroderma pigmentosum; hereditary retinoblastoma; CDKN2A mutation	Increase incidence	[27–31]	Probable evidence
Immune system deficiency/suppression	Increases incidence	[32,33]	Probable evidence
Previous radiotherapy	Increases incidence	[34,35]	Convincing evidence

Convincing evidence: good-quality studies, that is, metaanalyses, support this argument; epidemiological numbers are also considered convincing evidence (i.e., white race).
Probable evidence: few studies support the argument, or the results of relevant studies are contradictory.
BMI, Body mass index.

brain before the age of 20 years, with no significant effect of CT scans of other anatomical sites.

Table 2.2 summarizes in a parsimonious and easy manner the most probable risk factors for melanoma. An arbitrary dichotomous classification (convincing or probable evidence) was used, to spare the need of reporting numbers or study types. Items supported by convincing evidence are very unlikely to have an effect in the opposite direction than reported. Those marked probable are also not anticipated to change direction of the effect in the future but further studies are required.

References

[1] Mestnik NC, Afonso JP, et al. Melanoma developed during pregnancy—a case report. An Bras Dermatol 2014;89(1):157–9.
[2] Kyrgidis A. Risk factors for non-melanoma skin cancer. In: Maibach H, Gorouchi F, editors. Evidence based dermatology. North Carolina: PMH Publishers; 2010. p. 847–74.
[3] Bataille V, de Vries E. Melanoma—part 1: epidemiology, risk factors, and prevention. BMJ 2008;337:a2249.
[4] Guy GP Jr, Thomas CC, et al. Vital signs: melanoma incidence and mortality trends and projections—United States, 1982–2030. MMWR Morb Mortal Wkly Rep 2015;64(21):591–6.
[5] Khosrotehrani K, Dasgupta P, et al. Melanoma survival is superior in females across all tumour stages but is influenced by age. Arch Dermatol Res 2015;307(8):731–40.
[6] Stewart LM, Holman CD, et al. Association between in-vitro fertilization, birth and melanoma. Melanoma Res 2013;23(6):489–95.

[7] Wiren S, Haggstrom C, et al. Pooled cohort study on height and risk of cancer and cancer death. Cancer Causes Control 2014;25(2):151–9.

[8] Sergentanis TN, Antoniadis AG, et al. Obesity and risk of malignant melanoma: a meta-analysis of cohort and case–control studies. Eur J Cancer 2013;49(3):642–57.

[9] Gandini S, Sera F, et al. Meta-analysis of risk factors for cutaneous melanoma: I. Common and atypical naevi. Eur J Cancer 2005;41(1):28–44.

[10] Gandini S, Sera F, et al. Meta-analysis of risk factors for cutaneous melanoma: II. Sun exposure. Eur J Cancer 2005;41(1):45–60.

[11] Gandini S, Sera F, et al. Meta-analysis of risk factors for cutaneous melanoma: III. Family history, actinic damage and phenotypic factors. Eur J Cancer 2005;41(14):2040–59.

[12] Cho E, Rosner BA, et al. Risk factors and individual probabilities of melanoma for whites. J Clin Oncol 2005;23(12):2669–75.

[13] Rivers JK. Is there more than one road to melanoma? Lancet 2004;363(9410):728–30.

[14] Strouse JJ. Pediatric melanoma: risk factor and survival analysis of the surveillance, epidemiology and end results database. J Clin Oncol 2005;23(21):4735–41.

[15] Boniol M, Autier P, et al. Cutaneous melanoma attributable to sunbed use: systematic review and meta-analysis. BMJ 2012;345:e4757.

[16] Colantonio S, Bracken MB, et al. The association of indoor tanning and melanoma in adults: systematic review and meta-analysis. J Am Acad Dermatol 2014;70(5):847–57. e818.

[17] Elwood JM, Jopson J. Melanoma and sun exposure: an overview of published studies. Int J Cancer 1997;73(2):198–203.

[18] Autier P, Boniol M, et al. Sunscreen use and increased duration of intentional sun exposure: still a burning issue. Int J Cancer 2007;121(1):1–5.

[19] Chesnut C, Kim J. Is there truly no benefit with sunscreen use and basal cell carcinoma? A critical review of the literature and the application of new sunscreen labeling rules to real-world sunscreen practices. J Skin Cancer 2012;2012:1–4.

[20] Dennis LK, Beane Freeman LE, et al. Sunscreen use and the risk for melanoma: a quantitative review. Ann Intern Med 2003;139(12):966–78.

[21] Diffey B. Climate change, ozone depletion and the impact on ultraviolet exposure of human skin. Phys Med Biol 2003;49(1):R1–11.

[22] Diffey BL. A quantitative estimate of melanoma mortality from ultraviolet A sunbed use in the U.K.. Br J Dermatol 2003;149(3):578–81.

[23] Weinstock MA. Do sunscreens increase or decrease melanoma risk: an epidemiologic evaluation. J Investig Dermatol Symp Proc 1999;4(1):97–100.

[24] Olsen CM, Carroll HJ, et al. Estimating the attributable fraction for melanoma: a meta-analysis of pigmentary characteristics and freckling. Int J Cancer 2010;127(10):2430–45.

[25] Olsen CM, Carroll HJ, et al. Familial melanoma: a meta-analysis and estimates of attributable fraction. Cancer Epidemiol Biomarkers Prev 2010;19(1):65–73.

[26] Fallah M, Pukkala E, et al. Familial melanoma by histology and age: joint data from five Nordic countries. Eur J Cancer 2014;50(6):1176–83.

[27] Bishop DT. Geographical variation in the penetrance of CDKN2A mutations for melanoma. J Natl Cancer Inst 2002;94(12):894–903.

[28] Bonadies DC, Bale AE. Hereditary melanoma. Curr Probl Cancer 2011;35(4):162–72.

[29] Eng C, Li FP, et al. Mortality from second tumors among long-term survivors of retinoblastoma. J Natl Cancer Inst 1993;85(14):1121–8.

[30] Fletcher O, Easton D, et al. Lifetime risks of common cancers among retinoblastoma survivors. J Natl Cancer Inst 2004;96(5):357–63.

[31] Moll AC, Imhof SM, et al. Second primary tumors in patients with hereditary retinoblastoma: a register-based follow-up study, 1945–1994. Int J Cancer 1996;67(4):515–9.

[32] Lee MS, Lin RY, et al. The risk of developing non-melanoma skin cancer, lymphoma and melanoma in patients with psoriasis in Taiwan: a 10-year, population-based cohort study. Int J Dermatol 2012;51(12):1454–60.

[33] Singh S, Nagpal SJ, et al. Inflammatory bowel disease is associated with an increased risk of melanoma: a systematic review and meta-analysis. Clin Gastroenterol Hepatol 2014;12(2):210–8.
[34] Mathews JD, Forsythe AV, et al. Cancer risk in 680 000 people exposed to computed tomography scans in childhood or adolescence: data linkage study of 11 million Australians. BMJ 2013;346:f2360.
[35] Parkin DM, Darby SC. 12. Cancers in 2010 attributable to ionising radiation exposure in the UK. Br J Cancer 2011;105:S57–65.

Further Reading

Andtbacka RH, Donaldson MR, et al. Sentinel lymph node biopsy for melanoma in pregnant women. Ann Surg Oncol 2013;20(2):689–96.
Health issues of ultraviolet tanning appliances used for cosmetic purposes. Health Phys 2003;84(1):119–27.
Astner S, Anderson RR. Skin phototypes 2003. J Invest Dermatol 2004;122(2). xxx–xxxi.
Balch CM, Houghton AN, et al. Cutaneous melanoma, 4th edition. Dermatol Surg 2005;31(12):1715.
Balmer A, Zografos L, et al. Diagnosis and current management of retinoblastoma. Oncogene 2006;25(38):5341–9.
Bastuji-Garin S, Diepgen TL. Cutaneous malignant melanoma, sun exposure, and sunscreen use: epidemiological evidence. Br J Dermatol 2002;146(s61):24–30.
Bataille V, Boniol M, et al. A multicentre epidemiological study on sunbed use and cutaneous melanoma in Europe. Eur J Cancer 2005;41(14):2141–9.
Bataille V, Kato BS, et al. Nevus size and number are associated with telomere length and represent potential markers of a decreased senescence in vivo. Cancer Epidemiol Biomarkers Prev 2007;16(7):1499–502.
Bauer J, Garbe C. Acquired melanocytic nevi as risk factor for melanoma development. A comprehensive review of epidemiological data. Pigment Cell Res 2003;16(3):297–306.
Bauer A, Diepgen TL, et al. Is occupational solar ultraviolet irradiation a relevant risk factor for basal cell carcinoma? A systematic review and meta-analysis of the epidemiological literature. Br J Dermatol 2011;165:612–25.
Bennett DC. Human melanocyte senescence and melanoma susceptibility genes. Oncogene 2003;22(20):3063–9.
Birch JM, Alston RD, et al. Relative frequency and morphology of cancers in carriers of germline TP53 mutations. Oncogene 2001;20(34):4621–8.
Cleaver JE. Opinion: cancer in xeroderma pigmentosum and related disorders of DNA repair. Nat Rev Cancer 2005;5(7):564–73.
Coelho SG, Hearing VJ. UVA tanning is involved in the increased incidence of skin cancers in fair-skinned young women. Pigment Cell Melanoma Res 2009;23(1):57–63.
Cogliano VJ, Baan R, et al. Preventable exposures associated with human cancers. J Natl Cancer Inst 2011;103(24):1827–39.
Cokkinides V, Weinstock M, et al. Indoor tanning use among adolescents in the US, 1998 to 2004. Cancer 2008;115(1):190–8.
Cust AE, Armstrong BK, et al. Sunbed use during adolescence and early adulthood is associated with increased risk of early-onset melanoma. Int J Cancer 2010;128(10):2425–35.
Dahlke E, Murray CA, et al. Systematic review of melanoma incidence and prognosis in solid organ transplant recipients. Transplant Res 2014;3:10.
Dennis LK, Vanbeek MJ, et al. Sunburns and risk of cutaneous melanoma: does age matter? A comprehensive meta-analysis. Ann Epidemiol 2008;18(8):614–27.
Dulon M, Weichenthal M, et al. Sun exposure and number of nevi in 5- to 6-year-old European children. J Clin Epidemiol 2002;55(11):1075–81.

Ferrone CR. Clinicopathological features of and risk factors for multiple primary melanomas. JAMA 2005;294(13):1647.

Ferrucci LM, Cartmel B, et al. Indoor tanning and risk of early-onset basal cell carcinoma. J Am Acad Dermatol 2012;67(4):552–62.

Forsea AM, del Marmol V, et al. Melanoma incidence and mortality in Europe: new estimates, persistent disparities. Br J Dermatol 2012;167(5):1124–30.

Gallagher RP, Spinelli JJ, et al. Tanning beds, sunlamps, and risk of cutaneous malignant melanoma. Cancer Epidemiol Biomarkers Prev 2005;14(3):562–6.

Gerstenblith MR, Shi J, et al. Genome-wide association studies of pigmentation and skin cancer: a review and meta-analysis. Pigment Cell Melanoma Res 2010;23(5):587–606.

Gerstenblith MR, Rajaraman P, et al. Basal cell carcinoma and anthropometric factors in the U.S. radiologic technologists cohort study. Int J Cancer 2012;131(2):E149–55.

Goldenberg A, Vujic I, et al. Melanoma risk perception and prevention behavior among African-Americans: the minority melanoma paradox. Clin Cosmet Investig Dermatol 2015;8:423–9.

Hansen CB, Wadge LM, et al. Clinical germline genetic testing for melanoma. Lancet Oncol 2004;5(5):314–9.

Hussein MR. Melanocytic dysplastic naevi occupy the middle ground between benign melanocytic naevi and cutaneous malignant melanomas: emerging clues. J Clin Pathol 2005;58(5):453–6.

Kiiski V, de Vries E, et al. Risk factors for single and multiple basal cell carcinomas. Arch Dermatol 2010;146(8):848–55.

Kyrgidis A, Tzellos TG, Triaridis S. Melanoma: stem cells, sun exposure and hallmarks for carcinogenesis, molecular concepts and future clinical implications. J Carcinog 2010;9:3.

Law MH, MacGregor S, et al. Melanoma genetics: recent findings take us beyond well-traveled pathways. J Investig Dermatol 2012;132(7):1763–74.

Lazovich D, Vogel RI, et al. Indoor tanning and risk of melanoma: a case–control study in a highly exposed population. Cancer Epidemiol Biomarkers Prev 2010;19(6):1557–68.

Merlino G, Noonan FP. Modeling gene–environment interactions in malignant melanoma. Trends Mol Med 2003;9(3):102–8.

Naeyaert JM, Brochez L. Dysplastic nevi. N Engl J Med 2003;349(23):2233–40.

Nichols KE, Malkin D, et al. Germ-line p53 mutations predispose to a wide spectrum of early-onset cancers. Cancer Epidemiol Biomarkers Prev 2001;10(2):83–7.

Olivier M, Goldgar DE, et al. Li–Fraumeni and related syndromes: correlation between tumor type, family structure, and TP53 genotype. Cancer Res 2003;63(20):6643–50.

Olsen CM, Green AC, et al. Anthropometric factors and risk of melanoma in women: a pooled analysis. Int J Cancer 2007;122(5):1100–8.

Olsen CM, Zens MS, et al. Biologic markers of sun exposure and melanoma risk in women: pooled case–control analysis. Int J Cancer 2010;129(3):713–23.

Olsen CM, Knight LL, et al. Risk of melanoma in people with HIV/AIDS in the pre- and post-HAART eras: a systematic review and meta-analysis of cohort studies. PLoS One 2014;9(4):e95096.

Perry PK, Silverberg NB. Cutaneous malignancy in albinism. Cutis 2001;67(5):427–30.

Pfeifer GP, Besaratinia A. UV wavelength-dependent DNA damage and human non-melanoma and melanoma skin cancer. Photochem Photobiol Sci 2012;11(1):90–7.

Pfeifer GP, You YH, et al. Mutations induced by ultraviolet light. Mutat Res 2005;571(1–2):19–31.

Renehan AG, Tyson M, et al. Body-mass index and incidence of cancer: a systematic review and meta-analysis of prospective observational studies. Lancet 2008;371(9612):569–78.

Schmitt J, Seidler A, et al. Occupational ultraviolet light exposure increases the risk for the development of cutaneous squamous cell carcinoma: a systematic review and meta-analysis. Br J Dermatol 2011;164(2):291–307.

Tucker MA, Goldstein AM. Melanoma etiology: where are we? Oncogene 2003;22(20):3042–52.

Varley JM. Germline TP53 mutations and Li–Fraumeni syndrome. Hum Mutat 2003;21(5):551.

Vogel RI, Ahmed RL, et al. Exposure to indoor tanning without burning and melanoma risk by sunburn history. J Natl Cancer Inst 2014;106(7):dju219.

Wachsmuth RC, Gaut RM, et al. Heritability and gene–environment interactions for melanocytic nevus density examined in a U.K. adolescent twin study. J Invest Dermatol 2001;117(2):348–52.

Wehner MR, Shive ML, et al. Indoor tanning and non-melanoma skin cancer: systematic review and meta-analysis. BMJ 2012;345:e5909.

Williams PF, Olsen CM, et al. Melanocortin 1 receptor and risk of cutaneous melanoma: a meta-analysis and estimates of population burden. Int J Cancer 2011;129(7):1730–40.

Yamaguchi Y, Takahashi K, et al. Human skin responses to UV radiation: pigment in the upper epidermis protects against DNA damage in the lower epidermis and facilitates apoptosis. FASEB J 2006;20(9):1486–8.

Diagnosis of Primary Melanoma

Cutaneous Melanoma. http://dx.doi.org/10.1016/B978-0-12-804000-3.00003-X

SUBCHAPTER

3.1

Clinical Presentation

Aimilios Lallas*, Gabriella Brancaccio**

*Aristotle University of Thessaloniki, Thessaloniki, Greece
**University of Campania Luigi Vanvitelli, Naples, Italy

The melanoma family encompasses tumors with different clinical characteristics and biological behavior. In the current chapter, the selected classification is clinically oriented, aiming to follow the real scenarios that clinicians are faced with in their everyday practice.

1 CONVENTIONAL MELANOMA

It originates from melanocytes at the dermoepidermal junction and is initially restricted within the epidermis (melanoma in situ) growing mainly peripherally. After a period that ranges between few months and many years, it invades the dermis and acquires a significant metastatic potential [1].

The clinical characteristics and the differential diagnosis of CM largely depend on body location and can be subclassified as following:

1. Melanoma of the trunk and the extremities (superficial spreading melanoma: the most frequent clinical subtype)
2. Facial melanoma [lentigo maligna (LM) melanoma]
3. Acral melanoma (or acral lentiginous melanoma)
4. Nail melanoma
5. Mucosal melanoma
6. Primary extracutaneous melanoma, including ocular, CNS, and soft tissue melanoma

1.1 Melanoma of the Trunk and the Extremities

- Look for:
  - Light-to-dark brown or black flat macule (Fig. 3.1.1)

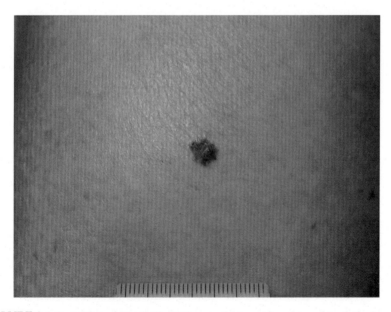

FIGURE 3.1.1   **Melanoma typically begins as a brown-colored macule, relatively symmetric in terms of shape and color distribution.**

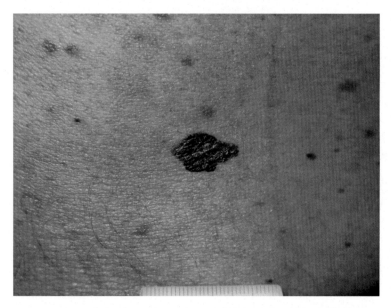

FIGURE 3.1.2 **With time, melanoma acquires the ABCD clinical criteria, showing asymmetry of shape, an abrupt border, more than one color, and a large diameter.**

- With time, development of a palpable elevated or papular component, appearance of multiple colors, shape and border irregularity (Fig. 3.1.2).
- Development of a nodular part, ulceration, or bleeding at a later stage (Fig. 3.1.3).
- If left untreated, invasion of the deeper and surrounding tissues by melanoma, resulting in an impressive clinical appearance [2].
- Differential diagnosis:
  - Nevi: Naturally symmetric (even when they increase in size), uniform in color, and with regular border:
    - Morphologically atypical nevi do exist (e.g., patients with the so-called "atypical mole syndrome"). In such cases, an accurate diagnosis is impossible without coupling clinical examination with dermoscopy [3].
  - Seborrheic keratosis (SK): "Stuck-on" appearance and sharp demarcation. Not uncommon color variegations [4].
  - Pigmented BCC: Might be very difficult to discriminate from melanoma. An elevated border and a translucent hue are in favor of pigmented BCC [5,6] (Fig. 3.1.4).
- Diagnostic pearls: The clinical criteria of melanoma have been summarized in the so-called ABCD clinical rule (Table 3.1.1).
- Management: Any lesion displaying the ABCD clinical criteria should be excised to rule out melanoma. The only exception to this rule is if dermoscopy reveals a clear-cut SK (Fig. 3.1.4).

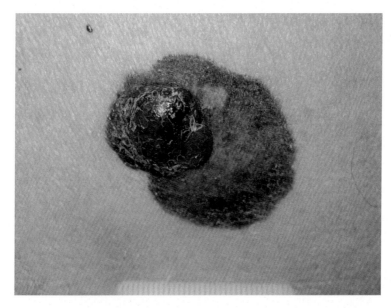

FIGURE 3.1.3 **At a later stage, the morphologic asymmetry is obvious, while a nodular part often develops, which might ulcerate or bleed.**

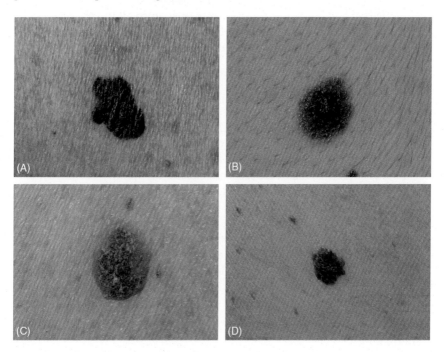

FIGURE 3.1.4 The main differential diagnosis of melanoma (A): nevus (B) which is typically symmetric in shape and, even if displaying a darker area, this is distributed "regularly" (in this example in the center). Seborrheic keratosis (C), which is characterized by a papillomatous surface and a "stuck-on" appearance. Pigmented basal cell carcinoma (D) might be very difficult to discriminate from melanoma on clinical grounds.

TABLE 3.1.1   The ABCD Clinical Rule for Melanoma Detection

A	Asymmetry
B	Border irregularity
C	Color variegation
D	Diameter >6 mm
(E)	Evolution

1.2 Facial Melanoma

- Overview:
  - Melanoma, LM, and LMM should be considered synonyms (or LM for melanoma in situ and LMM for invasive tumors).
  - Characterized by a slow lentiginous growth pattern, it represents the less aggressive melanoma subtype [1] (LM often remains for years or decades in situ).
- Look for:
  - A long-standing tan macule slowly expanding peripherally
  - Change in color (light brown, dark brown, and black areas) with time
  - Regression (whitish areas within the lesion):
    - When LM becomes invasive, it may acquire all the characteristics of invasive melanoma (asymmetry, irregularity of shape and border, development of papular/nodular part, ulceration, bleeding) (Fig. 3.1.5) [2].
- Differential diagnosis:
  - Nonmelanocytic tumors: Pigmented actinic keratosis (PAK) and solar lentigo (SL)/SK [7]:
    - The discrimination among LM, PAK, and SL/SK represents one of the most challenging clinical scenarios, even after dermoscopic examination (Fig. 3.1.6) [8,9].
    - Nevi on the face of elderly individuals are mainly dermal and elevated, not being included, thus, in the differential diagnosis of flat pigmented facial lesions [10].
- Diagnostic pearls:
  - The association with chronic sun exposure is stronger for LM than for any other subtype of melanoma. LM typically develops on heavily sun-damaged skin of elderly individuals, mainly on the face but also on the extremities [11].

1.3 Acral Melanoma

- Look for:
  - A pigmented flat lesion with variable shades of brown or black color
  - Irregular shape and multiple colors with growth (diameter more than 6–7 mm)

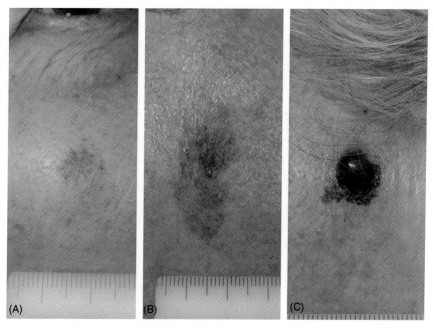

FIGURE 3.1.5 **Facial melanoma (lentigo maligna).** At an early stage (A) it presents as a clinically inconspicuous tan macule. Later (B), different shades of brown (or black) color often appear. At an advanced stage (C) a nodular component might develop.

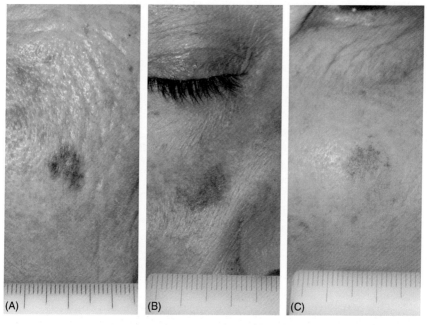

FIGURE 3.1.6 The differential diagnosis of facial melanoma (A) includes pigmented actinic keratosis (B) and solar lentigo/early seborrheic keratosis (C). As highlighted by this figure, the clinical discrimination among these entities is highly problematic.

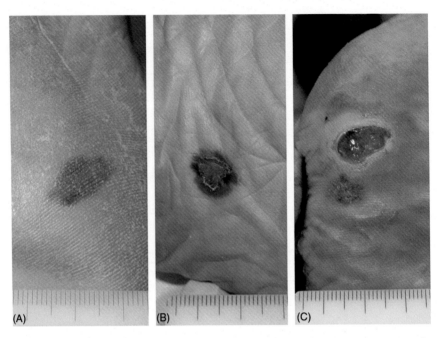

FIGURE 3.1.7   Early acral melanoma (A) presenting as a light brown symmetric macule. At this stage, the diagnosis without dermoscopy is very difficult. Later (B) an asymmetry of shape, an irregularity of border, and darker areas may appear. Advanced tumors (C) might ulcerate or bleed.

- Papular or nodular component, ulceration, or bleeding in more advanced tumors (Fig. 3.1.7) [12,13]:
  - AM develops much more frequently on the soles, as compared to on the palms [14].
- Differential diagnosis:
  - Acral nevi: Smaller, with a diameter not exceeding 7 mm, and characterized by a uniform light brown, dark brown, or black color and a regular shape [15,16]
  - Subcorneal hemorrhage: Sharp demarcation and resolution by scratching the epidermal surface
  - Viral warts or diabetic ulcers [17]

1.4 Nail Melanoma

- Overview:
  - Originates from melanocytes of the nail matrix and clinically develops as a pigmented nail band (longitudinal melanonychia)

- Look for:
    - A thin linear band of light brown, dark brown, or black color
    - Initially appearing at the proximal nail fold and gradually linearly expanding to the distal nail fold
    - With progression, increasing in thickness and losing the uniform hue (development of sequential bands of different shades of brown or black color):
        - The band gradually acquires a triangular shape, with its basis (thicker part) on the proximal fold and its top (thinner part) on the distal, reflecting the rapid growth of the melanoma of the nail matrix.
    - Invasion of the entire nail plate, onychodystrophia, ulceration, or bleeding at advanced stage
    - "Hutchinson's sign": Involvement of the proximal nail fold (Fig. 3.1.8)
- Differential diagnosis:
    - Subungual nevi are also present as longitudinal melanonychia, but they typically develop earlier in life, remain uniform in color, and do not usually cover large parts of the nail plate:
        - Congenital nevi represent an exception, since they may cover all the surface of the nail bed and also expand to the surrounding skin.
    - Reactive pigmentation
    - Subungual hemorrhage
    - Onychomycosis [18,19]

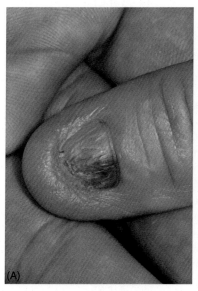 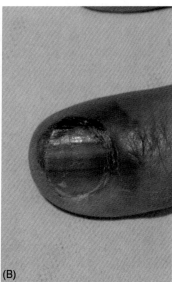

FIGURE 3.1.8 Nail melanoma (A) develops as a pigmented nail band and might cause onychodystrophy. With tumor progression (B), all the surface of the nail, as well as the surrounding skin, might be affected.

1.5 Mucosal Melanoma

- Overview:
  - Primary melanoma of the mucous membranes is a rare condition and may affect the lips, the gingiva or palate, the nasal mucosa, the vulva, or the glans penis.
- Look for:
  - A flat pigmented macule (even if this melanoma is often diagnosed at a late stage when it becomes nodular, asymmetric in shape and color, and ulcerated or bleeding)
- Differential diagnosis:
  - Benign melanotic macules, but also nevi, vascular tumors, and inflammatory and infectious diseases [20,21]

2 NODULAR MELANOMA

- Overview:
  - Less frequent but much more aggressive biologically; may metastasize from a very early stage, through either the lymphatic or the vascular pathway
- Look for:
  - A small papule rapidly enlarging into a nodule, which later might ulcerate or bleed
  - Symmetric in shape, well demarcated, and uniform in color, which might be black, blue, or pink/red (amelanotic NM):
    - The head/neck area, the trunk, and the extremities are the most frequent body locations [22].
- Differential diagnosis:
  - Dermal and blue nevus, hemangioma, pyogenic granuloma, angiokeratoma, SK, and other rare neoplasms [23]:
    - A very rare and extremely difficult to recognize type of NM is verrucous melanoma that might perfectly mimic benign tumors with a verrucous surface [24] (Fig. 3.1.9).
- Diagnostic pearls:
  - The ABCD clinical rule is completely inefficient in this case. The EFG clinical criteria are more appropriate, since they reflect the three main characteristics of NM: an *e*levated lesion of *f*irm consistency, which *g*rows rapidly (Table 3.1.2) [22,25].
    - Because of its clinical characteristics described previously, NM often escapes detection until progressing in an advanced stage (Fig. 3.1.9). In addition, NM often develops in "low-risk" individuals (i.e., with a low nevus count, without family history, etc.) [26].

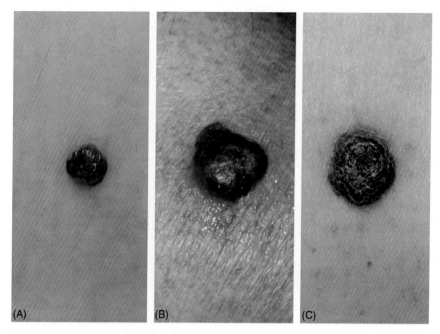

FIGURE 3.1.9 Nodular melanoma initially develops as a perfectly symmetric tumor that lacks the ABCD clinical criteria. (A) Often it is diagnosed only at an advanced stage (B) after the appearance of multiple colors, ulceration, or bleeding. Verrucous melanoma (C) is a rare variant that mimics benign keratinizing tumors.

TABLE 3.1.2   The EFG Clinical Rule for Nodular Melanoma

E	Elevated tumor
F	Firm consistency
G	Rapid growth

3 AMELANOTIC MELANOMA

- Overview:
  - AM does not represent a distinct melanoma subtype, since a proportion of both, CM and NM, are minimally or not at all pigmented.
- Look for:
  - A flat tumor with a whitish to pinkish or flesh-colored hue and shiny surface (flat AM)
  - Amelanotic from the very beginning or, more frequently, the lack of pigment representing a result of extensive regression
  - Rapidly growing pink or red nodule (nodular AM)

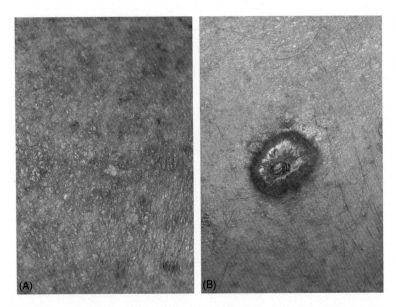

FIGURE 3.1.10   Flat amelanotic melanoma (A) displays very subtle clinical characteristics, rendering its clinical recognition extremely difficult. Nodular amelanotic melanoma (B) is also characterized by an unspecific clinical appearance and has to be differentiated mainly from basal cell carcinoma and vascular tumors.

- Differential diagnosis:
  - Superficial basal cell carcinoma, in situ squamous cell carcinoma, regressed nevus, and lichen planus-like keratosis (regressed SL or SK) [27] for flat AM
  - Basal cell carcinoma, squamous cell carcinoma, Merkel cell carcinoma, vascular tumors, and other less frequent neoplasms for nodular AM [23,28] (Fig. 3.1.10)

References

[1] Ackerman AB, David KM. A unifying concept of malignant melanoma: biologic aspects. Hum Pathol 1986;17:438–40.
[2] Rigel DS, Russak J, Friedman R. The evolution of melanoma diagnosis: 25 years beyond the ABCDs. CA Cancer J Clin 2010;60:301–16.
[3] Argenziano G, Catricalà C, Ardigo M, et al. Dermoscopy of patients with multiple nevi: improved management recommendations using a comparative diagnostic approach. Arch Dermatol 2011;147:46–9.
[4] Gill D, Dorevitch A, Marks R. The prevalence of seborrheic keratoses in people aged 15 to 30 years: is the term senile keratosis redundant? Arch Dermatol 2000;136:759–62.
[5] Scrivener Y, Grosshans E, Cribier B. Variations of basal cell carcinomas according to gender, age, location and histopathological subtype. Br J Dermatol 2002;147:41–7.

[6] Altamura D, Menzies SW, Argenziano G, et al. Dermatoscopy of basal cell carcinoma: morphologic variability of global and local features and accuracy of diagnosis. J Am Acad Dermatol 2010;62:67–75.

[7] Schiffner R, Schiffner-Rohe J, Vogt T, et al. Improvement of early recognition of lentigo maligna using dermatoscopy. J Am Dermatol 2000;42:25–32.

[8] Pock L, Drlík L, Hercogová J. Dermatoscopy of pigmented actinic keratosis—a striking similarity to lentigo maligna. Int J Dermatol 2007;46(4):414–6.

[9] Zalaudek I, Ferrara G, Leinweber B, Mercogliano A, D'Ambrosio A, Argenziano G. Pitfalls in the clinical and dermoscopic diagnosis of pigmented actinic keratosis. J Am Acad Dermatol 2005;53:1071–4.

[10] Zalaudek I, Schmid K, Marghoob AA, et al. Frequency of dermoscopic nevus subtypes by age and body site: a cross-sectional study. Arch Dermatol 2011;147:663–70.

[11] Tiodorovic-Zivkovic D, Argenziano G, Lallas A, et al. Age, gender, and topography influence the clinical and dermoscopic appearance of lentigo maligna. J Am Acad Dermatol 2015;72:801–8.

[12] Saida T. Malignant melanoma on the sole: how to detect the early lesions efficiently. Pigment Cell Res 2000;13(Suppl. 8):135–9.

[13] Saida T, Koga H. Dermoscopic patterns of acral melanocytic nevi: their variations, changes, and significance. Arch Dermatol 2007;143:1423–6.

[14] Lallas A, Sgouros D, Zalaudek I, et al. Palmar and plantar melanomas differ for sex prevalence and tumor thickness but not for dermoscopic patterns. Melanoma Res 2014;24:83–7.

[15] Saida T, Koga H, Uhara H. Key points in dermoscopic differentiation between early acral melanoma and acral nevus. J Dermatol 2011;38:25–34.

[16] Oguchi S, Saida T, Koganehira Y, Ohkubo S, Ishihara Y, Kawachi S. Characteristic epiluminescent microscopic features of early malignant melanoma on glabrous skin. A videomicroscopic analysis. Arch Dermatol 1998;134:563–8.

[17] Dalmau J, Abellaneda C, Puig S, Zaballos P, Malvehy J. Acral melanoma simulating warts: dermoscopic clues to prevent missing a melanoma. Dermatol Surg 2006;32:1072–8.

[18] Braun RP, Baran R, Le Gal F-A, et al. Diagnosis and management of nail pigmentations. J Am Acad Dermatol 2007;56:835–47.

[19] Piraccini BM, Balestri R, Starace M, Rech G. Nail digital dermoscopy (onychoscopy) in the diagnosis of onychomycosis. J Eur Acad Dermatol Venerol 2011;27:509–13.

[20] Kato T, Takematsu H, Tomita Y, Takahashi M, Abe R. Malignant melanoma of mucous membranes. A clinicopathologic study of 13 cases in Japanese patients. Arch Dermatol 1987;123:216–20.

[21] Blum A. Dermoscopy of pigmented lesions of the mucosa and the mucocutaneous junction. Arch Dermatol 2011;147:1181.

[22] Chamberlain AJ, Fritschi L, Kelly JW. Nodular melanoma: patients' perceptions of presenting features and implications for earlier detection. J Am Dermatol 2003;48:694–701.

[23] Menzies SW, Moloney FJ, Byth K, et al. Dermoscopic evaluation of nodular melanoma. JAMA Dermatol 2013;149:699–709.

[24] Longo C, Moscarella E, Piana S, et al. Not all lesions with a verrucous surface are seborrheic keratoses. J Am Acad Dermatol 2014;70:e121–3.

[25] Argenziano G, Longo C, Cameron A, et al. Blue-black rule: a simple dermoscopic clue to recognize pigmented nodular melanoma. Br J Dermatol 2011;165:1251–5.

[26] Thomas NE, Kricker A, Waxweiler WT, et al. Comparison of clinicopathologic features and survival of histopathologically amelanotic and pigmented melanomas: a population-based study. JAMA Dermatol 2014;150:1306–14.

[27] Jaimes N, Braun RP, Thomas L, Marghoob AA. Clinical and dermoscopic characteristics of amelanotic melanomas that are not of the nodular subtype. J Eur Acad Dermatol Venereol 2012;26:591–6.

[28] Zalaudek I, Kreusch J, Giacomel J, Ferrara G, Catricalà C, Argenziano G. How to diagnose nonpigmented skin tumors: a review of vascular structures seen with dermoscopy: part II. Nonmelanocytic skin tumors. J Am Acad Dermatol 2010;63:377–86. [quiz 387–8].

Further Reading

Clark WH, Elder DE, Van Horn M. The biologic forms of malignant melanoma. Hum Pathol 1986;17:443–50.

Clark WH, From L, Bernardino EA, Mihm MC. The histogenesis and biologic behavior of primary human malignant melanomas of the skin. Cancer Res 1969;29:705–27.

McGovern VJ, Cochran AJ, Van der Esch EP, Little JH, MacLennan R. The classification of malignant melanoma, its histological reporting and registration: a revision of the 1972 Sydney classification. Pathology 1986;18:12–21.

Forman SB, Ferringer TC, Peckham SJ, et al. Is superficial spreading melanoma still the most common form of malignant melanoma? J Am Acad Dermatol 2008;58:1013–20.

Coit DG, Andtbacka R, Anker CJ, et al. Melanoma. J Natl Compr Canc Netw 2012;10:366–400.

Coit DG, Andtbacka R, Anker CJ, et al. Melanoma, version 2.2013: featured updates to the NCCN guidelines. J Natl Compr Canc Netw 2013;11:395–407.

Kanzler MH, Swetter SM. Malignant melanoma. J Am Acad Dermatol 2003;48:780–3.

Ackerman AB. Mythology and numerology in the sphere of melanoma. Cancer 2000;88: 491–6.

Koh HK, Michalik E, Sober AJ, et al. Lentigo maligna melanoma has no better prognosis than other types of melanoma. J Clin Oncol 1984;2:994–1001.

Rigel DS, Carucci JA. Malignant melanoma: prevention, early detection, and treatment in the 21st century. CA Cancer J Clin 2000;50:215–36. [quiz 237–40].

Friedman RJ, Rigel DS, Kopf AW. Early detection of malignant melanoma: the role of physician examination and self-examination of the skin. CA Cancer J Clin 1985;35:130–51.

Ishihara K, Saida T, Otsuka F, Yamazaki N. Prognosis and Statistical Investigation Committee of the Japanese Skin Cancer Society. Statistical profiles of malignant melanoma and other skin cancers in Japan: 2007 update. Int J Clin Oncol 2008;13:33–41.

Bradford PT, Goldstein AM, McMaster ML, Tucker MA. Acral lentiginous melanoma: incidence and survival patterns in the United States, 1986–2005. Arch Dermatol 2009;145:427–34.

Stevens NG, Liff JM, Weiss NS. Plantar melanoma: is the incidence of melanoma of the sole of the foot really higher in blacks than whites? Int J Cancer 1990;45:691–3.

Green AC, Baade P, Coory M, Aitken JF, Smithers M. Population-based 20-year survival among people diagnosed with thin melanomas in Queensland, Australia. J Clin Oncol 2012;30:1462–7.

Chi Z, Li S, Sheng X, et al. Clinical presentation, histology, and prognoses of malignant melanoma in ethnic Chinese: a study of 522 consecutive cases. BMC Cancer 2011;11:85.

3.2

Dermoscopy

Aimilios Lallas*, Gabriella Brancaccio**
*Aristotle University of Thessaloniki, Thessaloniki, Greece
**University of Campania Luigi Vanvitelli, Naples, Italy

Dermoscopy significantly improves the sensitivity and specificity of clinicians for melanoma diagnosis [1]: it allows the detection of clinically inconspicuous melanomas (earlier stages) and enables the recognition of benign lesions that might look clinically worrisome, reducing, thus, the number of unnecessary excisions [2].

The dermoscopic criteria of melanoma are a result of its asymmetric growth and vary among different subtypes of the disease.

1 CONVENTIONAL MELANOMA

1.1 Melanoma of the Trunk and the Extremities

- Look for:
  - Asymmetry of shape
  - More than two colors (light brown, dark brown, black, blue, gray, red, white)
  - Asymmetry of structures [3,4]:
    - Local dermoscopic features associated with melanoma are summarized and analytically described in Table 3.2.1 (Figs. 3.2.1 and 3.2.2).
- Diagnostic pearls:
  - The dermoscopic diagnosis of melanoma is usually straightforward, but in some cases an analytic approach of the lesion is required *(two-step algorithm) as follows*:
    - Classify the lesion as melanocytic or not:
      - Melanocytic: Presence of pigment network, globules, streaks, or homogenous pigmentation (as prominent feature) or absence of any specific criteria

TABLE 3.2.1   Dermoscopic Criteria of Melanoma

Criteria	Description
Atypical pigment network	Black, brown, or gray network with irregular holes and thick lines
Irregular blotch(es)	Black, brown, or gray structureless areas with asymmetric distribution within the lesion
Irregular dots/ globules	Black or brown, round to oval, variously sized structures, irregularly distributed within the lesion
Irregular streaks/ pseudopods	Radial lines with (pseudopods) or without (streaks) a bulbous projection at their peripheral ending, irregularly distributed at the periphery of the lesion. They may arise from network structures but more often do not. They range in color from tan to black
Regression structures	They correspond to a clinically flat part of the lesion and are of two kinds: 1. White scar-like depigmented areas 2. Blue-gray pepper-like granules
Blue-white veil	Structureless area of confluent blue color with an overlying white "ground-glass" film. The area cannot cover the entire surface of the lesion. It corresponds to a clinically elevated part
Atypical vascular pattern	1. Linear irregular vessels 2. Polymorphous vascular pattern consisting of dotted plus linear (of any kind) vessels

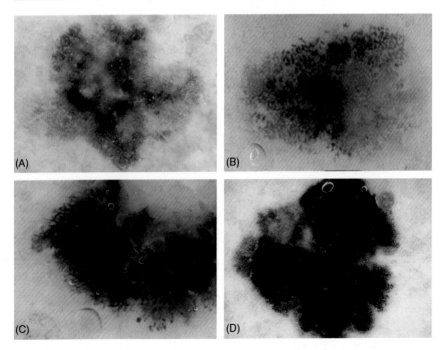

(A)   (B)

(C)   (D)

FIGURE 3.2.1   Examples of dermoscopic criteria of melanoma, defined in Table 3.2.1: (A) atypical network, (B) irregular globules, (C) irregular streaks/pseudopods, and (D) irregular blotches.

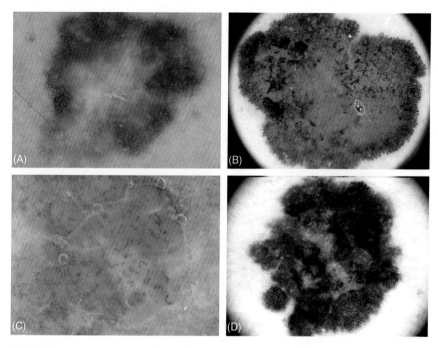

FIGURE 3.2.2 Examples of dermoscopic criteria of melanoma, defined in Table 3.2.1: (A) regression structures, (B) blue-white veil, and (C) atypical vascular pattern (linear irregular vessels). (D) A typical melanoma displaying several of the "classic" criteria, namely, atypical network, irregular dots, irregular blotches, and blue-white veil.

- Nonmelanocytic: Presence of criteria specifically associated with basal cell carcinoma, seborrheic keratosis (SK), or angioma
  - The first step of the algorithm is shown in Table 3.2.2.
- Differentiate melanoma from nevi [3,5–7]:
  - By pattern analysis (Table 3.2.3): Takes into account all the observed features (global and local), but without using any scoring system:
    - Not well reproducible and depending on the experience of the single clinician
  - By semiquantitative algorithms (the ABCD rule, the Menzies method, and the seven-point checklist) (Table 3.2.4):
    - It is simpler and easier to be used by nonexperts, and achieves similar results in terms of sensitivity but specificity is lower than that of pattern analysis.
    - It is not applicable to in situ and early invasive melanomas. Melanoma in situ usually displays subtle dermoscopic characteristics, such as atypical network alone or combined with areas of regression (Fig. 3.2.3) [8,9]. According to

TABLE 3.2.2   The First Step of the Two-Step Algorithm

Criteria suggestive of a melanocytic lesion	Criteria suggestive of a nonmelanocytic lesion
Pigment network	Milia-like cysts (SK)
Aggregated globules	Comedo-like openings (SK)
Streaks	Fingerprinting (SK)
Homogenous blue pigmentation	Brain-like appearance (SK)
	Arborizing vessels (BCC)
	Blue-gray ovoid nests (BCC)
	Multiple blue-gray globules (BCC)
	Leaf-like structures (BCC)
	Spoke wheel areas (BCC)
	Red/blue/black lacunas (angioma)
None of these criteria	

BCC, basal cell carcinoma; SK, seborrheic keratosis.

TABLE 3.2.3   The Second Step of the Two-Step Algorithm: Pattern Analysis

Criteria suggestive of nevus	Criteria suggestive of melanoma
Global patterns	
Reticular	Multicomponent
Globular	
Homogeneous	
Starburst	
Local features	
Typical pigment network (uniformly spaced holes and thin network lines)	Atypical pigment network (unequally spaced holes and thick network lines)
Regularly distributed dots/globules	Irregularly distributed dots/globules
Peripheral streaks symmetrically distributed	Peripheral streaks asymmetrically distributed
Central blotch	Eccentric blotch
Typical vascular pattern (comma vessels)	Blue-white veil
	Atypical vascular pattern (linear irregular vessels or polymorphous vessels)

TABLE 3.2.4   Second Step of the Two-Step Algorithm

ABCD rule		
A (asymmetry)	Asymmetry in zero, one, or two axes, regarding contour, color, and structures	Score 0–2
B (border)	Border abruptly interrupted at the periphery in zero to eight segments	Score 0–8
C (color)	Presence of up to six colors (white, red, light brown, dark brown, blue-gray, black)	Score 1–6
D (dermoscopic structures)	Presence of pigment network, dots, globules, streaks, structureless homogeneous areas	Score 1–5

Total dermoscopic score (TDS): (A × 1.3) + (B × 0.1) + (C × 0.5) + (D × 0.5)

Interpretation of TDS: <4.75, nevus; 4.75–5.45, suspicious lesion; >5.45, melanoma

Menzies method	
Negative features	**Positive features**
Symmetry of dermoscopic structures	Blue-white veil
Presence of a single color	Multiple brown dots
	Pseudopods
	Radial streaks
	Scar-like depigmentation
	Peripheral dots/globules
	Multiple (five or six) colors
	Multiple blue-gray dots
	Broadened network

Interpretation: A diagnosis of melanoma is made when both negative features are absent and one or more of the nine positive features are present

Seven-point checklist	
Dermoscopic features	**Score**
Major criteria	
1. Atypical pigment network	2
2. Blue-white veil	2
3. Atypical vascular pattern	2
Minor criteria	
4. Irregular streaks	1
5. Irregular dots and globules	1
6. Irregular blotches	1
7. Regression structures	1

Interpretation: Total score ≥3, melanoma; total score <3, nevus

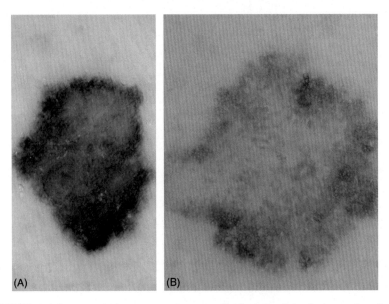

(A)   (B)

FIGURE 3.2.3   (A and B) In situ melanomas displaying subtle dermoscopic criteria, namely, atypical network combined with areas showing regression.

the "updated" version of the seven-point checklist, the presence of only one of the seven melanoma criteria should be considered enough to warrant excision [10].

1.2 Facial Melanoma

- Overview:
  - Melanocytic proliferations on the face (both benign and malignant) do not result in a dermoscopic pigment network, because of the relatively flattened dermoepidermal junction of the facial skin.
- Look for:
  - "Pseudonetwork" pattern: Structureless diffuse brown pigmentation, interrupted by numerous, variably broad hypopigmented holes, which correspond to hair follicles and sweat gland openings
    - Highly unspecific, since it can be seen in nevi, melanoma, and nonmelanocytic tumors [11]
- Diagnostic pearls (Table 3.2.5):
  - Gray circles/asymmetric follicular openings
  - Gray dots/globules (annular-granular pattern)
  - Rhomboidal structures [12,13]
  - Obliterated follicles (Fig. 3.2.4)
    - Gray color being the most frequent dermoscopic criterion of LM [14,15]
    - Vascular criteria also been described [16]

TABLE 3.2.5   Dermoscopic Criteria of Facial Melanoma (Lentigo Maligna Melanoma)

Dermoscopic criteria	
Pseudonetwork	White scar-like areas
Asymmetric pigmented follicular openings	Milky red areas
Slate gray dots	Increased density of the vascular network
Slate gray globules	Red rhomboidal structures
Rhomboidal structures	Target-like patterns
Annular-granular pattern	Darkening at dermoscopic examination
Gray-brown streaks	Circle within a circle
Dark/blue homogenous areas	Zigzag pattern

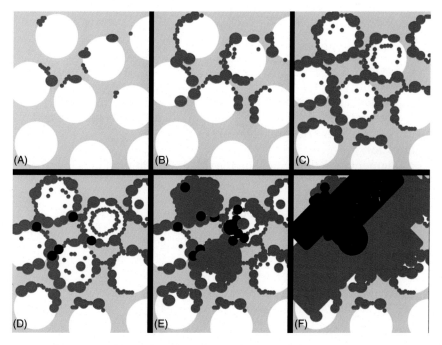

FIGURE 3.2.4   The dermoscopic progression model of facial melanoma (lentigo maligna): (A) gray dots/globules, (B) asymmetrically pigmented follicular openings, semicircles, (C) gray circles and gray rhomboidal structures, (D) circle within a circle, (E) obliterated follicles, and (F) structureless gray/brown/black areas.

- Differential diagnosis:
  - Pigmented actinic keratosis (PAK) [17,18]
  - Solar lentigo (SL)/early SK:
    - Table 3.2.6 shows the most useful features for the differential diagnosis of a facial pigmented macule.

TABLE 3.2.6   Useful Dermoscopic Structures for the Differential Diagnosis of a
Pigmented Facial Lesion

Lentigo maligna	Pigmented actinic keratosis	Solar lentigo/early seborrheic keratosis
Gray circles	Scales	Fingerprinting
Rhomboidal structures	White circles	Sharp demarcation
Obliterated follicles	Rosettes	Comedo-like openings
Circle within a circle	Evident follicles	Milia-like cysts
Brown/blue homogenous areas	Red color	Brain-like appearance
Zigzag pattern	Keratin plugs	Moth-eaten border

1.3 Acral Melanoma

- Overview:
  - Melanocytic proliferations on the acral skin do not dermoscopically display a pigment network, but an accentuation of the pigmentation along parallel skin markings: parallel furrows and ridges (pattern of parallel lines) [19,20].
- Look for:
  - Pigmentation distributed on the ridges of skin markings [parallel ridge pattern (PRP)].
- Differential diagnosis:
  - Nevi: pigmentation distributed along the epidermal furrows [parallel furrow pattern (PFP)] (Fig. 3.2.5) *or* others (fibrillar pattern, lattice-like pattern, double-line pattern) [20–23].
- Diagnostic pearls:
  - Ridges are much broader than furrows.
  - Always focus on the peripheral parts of the lesion.
  - Follow BRAAFF checklist (Table 3.2.7) [24].

1.4 Nail Melanoma

- Overview:
  - Melanocytic proliferations of the nail matrix clinically present as longitudinal melanonychia (melanonychia striata).
- Look for:
  - A pigmented band composed of parallel lines variable in the degree of pigmentation, thickness, and spacing (Fig. 3.2.6), and/or small brown granules.

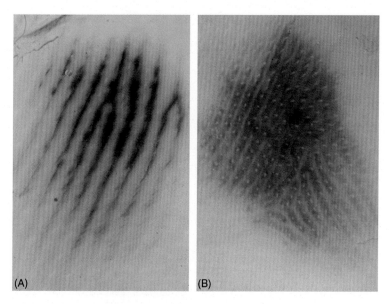

FIGURE 3.2.5 (A) Acral nevus: pigmentation follows the skin furrows, which are thinner than the ridges (parallel furrow pattern). In contrast, acral melanoma (B) is dermoscopically typified by a parallel ridge pattern of pigmentation.

TABLE 3.2.7 The BRAAFF Checklist for the Diagnosis of Acral Melanoma

Acronym	Criterion	Points
B	Irregular blotch	+1
R	Parallel ridge pattern	+3
A	Asymmetry of structures	+1
A	Asymmetry of colors	+1
F	Parallel furrow pattern	−1
F	Fibrillar pattern	−1

A score of 1 is needed for the diagnosis of melanoma.

- Differential diagnosis:
  - Nonmelanocytic melanonychias (hematoma, fungal infections): Homogenous distribution of pigment, sharp demarcation, interruption before the proximal nail fold [25,26].
  - Melanocytic nevi: Thinner band composed of parallel thin lines of similar brown hue with regular spacing among them:
    - Exception: Congenital nevi of the nail matrix might affect all the surface of the nail plate as well as the surrounding skin [25].
  - Subungual lentigo that usually reveals a grayish hue.

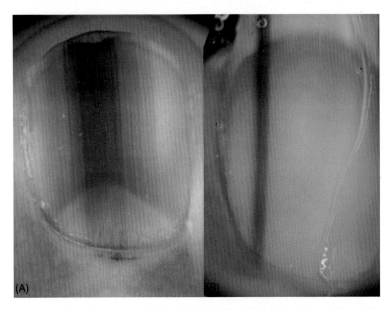

FIGURE 3.2.6   Melanonychia caused by melanoma (A) and nevus (B). The nail band in melanoma consists of parallel lines that vary in the degree of pigmentation, in their thickness and spacing. Furthermore, the nail band of melanoma is much wider as compared to the nevus band, which consists of parallel thin lines of similar brown hue with regular spacing among them.

1.5 Mucosal Melanoma

- Look for:
  - Structureless pattern
  - Gray, blue, or white color
- Differential diagnosis:
  - Nevi and benign melanotic macule: Light or dark brown coloration with pattern of lines or circles [27]

2 NODULAR MELANOMA

- Overview:
  - Most of the dermoscopic structures of conventional melanoma cannot be seen in nodular melanoma (NM). This is because they correspond to pigment deposition at the level of the dermoepidermal junction, while the neoplastic cells in NM are located within the dermis [28,29].
- Look for:
  - The simultaneous presence of blue and black color within the same lesion (blue-black rule) provided that the black color does

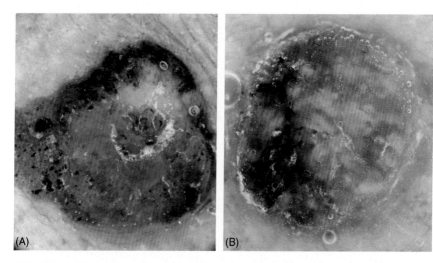

FIGURE 3.2.7 **Purely nodular melanomas lacking the classic melanoma criteria.** (A) The presence of blue and black color within the same lesion is highly suggestive of melanoma. (B) No specific melanoma criterion can be seen in this tumor. The only safe strategy for not to miss featureless nodular melanomas like this one is to excise all nodules that cannot be safely and specifically diagnosed by clinical and dermoscopic examination.

not correspond to clear-cut comedo-like openings (SK) or vascular lacunas (hemangiomas)
- An atypical vascular pattern, consisting of either linear irregular vessels or more than two morphologic types of vessels
- A pink (milky red) background color, even in the absence of any recognizable structure (Fig. 3.2.7) [28–30]
- Diagnostic pearls:
  - After clinical and dermoscopic examination, when a specific and confident diagnosis of a benign tumor (SK, hemangioma, dermal nevus or blue nevus) is not feasible, the lesion should be excised to rule out NM.

3 AMELANOTIC MELANOMA

- Overview:
  - In the absence of pigment, the only dermoscopic criteria remaining to be assessed are the vascular structures and the overall color hue.
- Look for:
  - Atypical vascular pattern
  - Pink (milky-red) color [29,30] (Fig. 3.2.8)

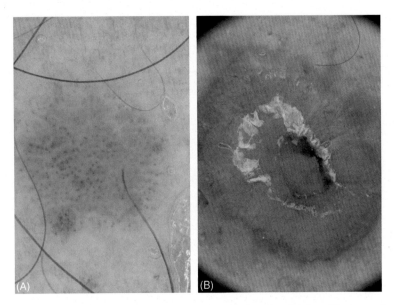

FIGURE 3.2.8 **Amelanotic melanomas do not display the classic melanoma criteria.**
(A) Dotted vessels might be the only detectable structure in flat amelanotic melanoma. (B)
A pinkish color and a polymorphous vascular pattern are highly predictive of a malignant
tumor, such as this amelanotic nodular melanoma.

- Differential diagnosis:
  - Melanocytic tumor (nevus or melanoma): dotted vessels:
    - Intraepidermal carcinoma (Bowen's disease) also displays
      dotted vessels, but they are usually larger in diameter and coiled
      (glomerular vessels) [31].
  - Basal cell carcinoma: Sharp in focus, linear vessels
  - Actinic keratosis: diffuse perifollicular erythema (strawberry
    pattern) [32]
  - Squamous cell carcinoma, Merkel cell carcinoma, atypical
    fibroxanthoma, and other uncommon malignancies [33,34]: Pink
    (milky-red) color and polymorphous vessels:
    - Given that a dermoscopic differentiation among these entities is
      impossible, and the fact that they all represent neoplasms with a
      considerable malignant potential, a tumor exhibiting this pattern
      should be undoubtedly excised.

References

[1] Vestergaard ME, Macaskill P, Holt PE, Menzies SW. Dermoscopy compared with naked
    eye examination for the diagnosis of primary melanoma: a meta-analysis of studies
    performed in a clinical setting. Br J Dermatol 2008;159:669–76.

[2] Argenziano G, Ferrara G, Francione S, Nola KD, Martino A, Zalaudek I. Dermoscopy—the ultimate tool for melanoma diagnosis. Semin Cutan Med Surg 2009;28:142–8.

[3] Argenziano G, Soyer HP, Chimenti S, et al. Dermoscopy of pigmented skin lesions: results of a consensus meeting via the internet. J Am Acad Dermatol 2003;48:679–93.

[4] Babino G, Lallas A, Longo C, Moscarella E, Alfano R, Argenziano G. Dermoscopy of melanoma and non-melanoma skin cancer. G Ital Dermatol Venereol 2015;150: 507–19.

[5] Nachbar F, Stolz W, Merkle T, et al. The ABCD rule of dermatoscopy. High prospective value in the diagnosis of doubtful melanocytic skin lesions. J Am Dermatol 1994;30: 551–9.

[6] Menzies SW, Ingvar C, Crotty KA, McCarthy WH. Frequency and morphologic characteristics of invasive melanomas lacking specific surface microscopic features. Arch Dermatol 1996;132:1178–82.

[7] Kittler H. Dermatoscopy: introduction of a new algorithmic method based on pattern analysis for diagnosis of pigmented skin lesions. Dermatopathol Practical Conceptual 2007;13:1.

[8] Argenziano G, Kittler H, Ferrara G, et al. Slow-growing melanoma: a dermoscopy follow-up study. Br J Dermatol 2010;162:267–73.

[9] Seidenari S, Bassoli S, Borsari S, et al. Variegated dermoscopy of in situ melanoma. Dermatology 2012;224:262–70.

[10] Argenziano G, Catricalà C, Ardigo M, et al. Seven-point checklist of dermoscopy revisited. Br J Dermatol 2011;164:785–90.

[11] Lallas A, Argenziano G, Moscarella E, Longo C, Simonetti V, Zalaudek I. Diagnosis and management of facial pigmented macules. Clin Dermatol 2014;32:94–100.

[12] Schiffner R, Schiffner-Rohe J, Vogt T, et al. Improvement of early recognition of lentigo maligna using dermatoscopy. J Am Dermatol 2000;42:25–32.

[13] Stolz W, Schiffner R, Burgdorf WHC. Dermatoscopy for facial pigmented skin lesions. Clin Dermatol 2002;20:276–8.

[14] Tiodorovic-Zivkovic D, Argenziano G, Lallas A, et al. Age, gender, and topography influence the clinical and dermoscopic appearance of lentigo maligna. J Am Acad Dermatol 2015;72:801–8.

[15] Tschandl P, Rosendahl C, Kittler H. Dermatoscopy of flat pigmented facial lesions. J Eur Acad Dermatol Venereol 2015;29:120–7.

[16] Pralong P, Bathelier E, Dalle S, Poulalhon N, Debarbieux S, Thomas L. Dermoscopy of lentigo maligna melanoma: report of 125 cases. Br J Dermatol 2012;167:280–7.

[17] Akay BN, Kocyigit P, Heper AO, Erdem C. Dermatoscopy of flat pigmented facial lesions: diagnostic challenge between pigmented actinic keratosis and lentigo maligna. Br J Dermatol 2010;163:1212–7.

[18] Zalaudek I, Ferrara G, Leinweber B, Mercogliano A, D'Ambrosio A, Argenziano G. Pitfalls in the clinical and dermoscopic diagnosis of pigmented actinic keratosis. J Am Acad Dermatol 2005;53:1071–4.

[19] Saida T, Koga H. Dermoscopic patterns of acral melanocytic nevi: their variations, changes, and significance. Arch Dermatol 2007;143:1423–6.

[20] Saida T, Koga H, Uhara H. Key points in dermoscopic differentiation between early acral melanoma and acral nevus. J Dermatol 2011;38:25–34.

[21] Saida T. Malignant melanoma on the sole: how to detect the early lesions efficiently. Pigment Cell Res 2000;13(Suppl. 8):135–9.

[22] Saida T, Miyazaki A, Oguchi S, et al. Significance of dermoscopic patterns in detecting malignant melanoma on acral volar skin: results of a multicenter study in Japan. Arch Dermatol 2004;140:1233–8.

[23] Oguchi S, Saida T, Koganehira Y, Ohkubo S, Ishihara Y, Kawachi S. Characteristic epiluminescent microscopic features of early malignant melanoma on glabrous skin. A videomicroscopic analysis. Arch Dermatol 1998;134:563–8.

[24] Lallas A, Kyrgidis A, Koga H, et al. The BRAAFF checklist: a new dermoscopic algorithm for diagnosing acral melanoma. Br J Dermatol 2015;173:1041–9.

[25] Braun RP, Baran R, Le Gal F-A, et al. Diagnosis and management of nail pigmentations. J Am Acad Dermatol 2007;56:835–47.

[26] Piraccini BM, Balestri R, Starace M, Rech G. Nail digital dermoscopy (onychoscopy) in the diagnosis of onychomycosis. J Eur Acad Dermatol Venerol 2011;27:509–13.

[27] Blum A. Dermoscopy of pigmented lesions of the mucosa and the mucocutaneous junction. Arch Dermatol 2011;147:1181.

[28] Argenziano G, Longo C, Cameron A, et al. Blue-black rule: a simple dermoscopic clue to recognize pigmented nodular melanoma. Br J Dermatol 2011;165:1251–5.

[29] Menzies SW, Moloney FJ, Byth K, et al. Dermoscopic evaluation of nodular melanoma. JAMA Dermatol 2013;149:699–709.

[30] Zalaudek I, Kreusch J, Giacomel J, Ferrara G, Catricalà C, Argenziano G. How to diagnose nonpigmented skin tumors: a review of vascular structures seen with dermoscopy: part II. Nonmelanocytic skin tumors. J Am Acad Dermatol 2010;63:377–86. [quiz 387–8].

[31] Zalaudek I, Argenziano G, Leinweber B, et al. Dermoscopy of Bowen's disease. Br J Dermatol 2004;150:1112–6.

[32] Jaimes N, Braun RP, Thomas L, Marghoob AA. Clinical and dermoscopic characteristics of amelanotic melanomas that are not of the nodular subtype. J Eur Acad Dermatol Venereol 2012;26:591–6.

[33] Lallas A, Pyne J, Kyrgidis A, et al. The clinical and dermoscopic features of invasive cutaneous squamous cell carcinoma depend on the histopathological grade of differentiation. Br J Dermatol 2014;172:1308–15.

[34] Lallas A, Moscarella E, Argenziano G, et al. Dermoscopy of uncommon skin tumours. Australas J Dermatol 2014;55:53–62.

Further Reading

Argenziano G, Fabbrocini G, Carli P, de Giorgi V, Sammarco E, Delfino M. Epiluminescence microscopy for the diagnosis of doubtful melanocytic skin lesions. Comparison of the ABCD rule of dermatoscopy and a new 7-point checklist based on pattern analysis. Arch Dermatol 1998;134:1563–70.

Argenziano G, Zalaudek I, Ferrara G, et al. Dermoscopy features of melanoma incognito: indications for biopsy. J Am Acad Dermatol 2007;56:508–13.

Lallas A, Zalaudek I, Apalla Z, et al. Management rules to detect melanoma. Dermatology 2013;226:52–60.

Lallas A, Sgouros D, Zalaudek I, et al. Palmar and plantar melanomas differ for sex prevalence and tumor thickness but not for dermoscopic patterns. Melanoma Res 2014;24:83–7.

Zaballos P, Blazquez S, Puig S, et al. Dermoscopic pattern of intermediate stage in seborrhoeic keratosis regressing to lichenoid keratosis: report of 24 cases. Br J Dermatol 2007;157:266–72.

3.3

Reflectance Confocal Microscopy

Caterina Longo

University of Modena and Reggio Emilia, Reggio Emilia, Italy

Reflectance confocal microscopy (RCM) is a relatively novel imaging technique that has been proved to improve the specificity for melanoma diagnosis when used as a second-level examination for dermoscopically difficult-to-diagnose lesions [1–3].

It is useful:

- To differentiate melanoma from nevi [1] (through an RCM score, based on six distinct morphologic features)
- In the case of facial lesions for which a biopsy is not always accepted by the patients and sufficient for the pathologist to make a conclusive diagnosis [3]

In this chapter we provide an overview of the different confocal morphologies of melanoma as a function of the anatomic location of the lesion.

1 BASIC PRINCIPLE AND INSTRUMENTS

- Two confocal microscopes are commercially available: a full-scale microscope constituted by a large scanning head (VivaScope 1500, Lucid Inc., Rochester, NY) and a handheld RCM (VivaScope 3000).
  - The handheld version is a smaller, flexible device quite useful in difficult-to-access areas or surgical premapping.
- The mechanism of bright contrast in RCM is backscattering.
  - Backscattering is primarily governed by the structures' refractive index compared to surrounding medium.
  - In gray-scale confocal images, structures that appear bright (white) have components with high refractive index compared with their surroundings and are similar in size to the wavelength of light.

- Highly reflective skin components include melanin, collagen, and keratin.
- The confocal scanning produces high-resolution black and white horizontal images (0.5×0.5 mm) with a lateral resolution of 1.0 µm and axial resolution of 3–5 µm.
- A sequence of full-resolution individual images at a given depth is acquired and "stitched" together to create a mosaic ranging in size from 2×2 to 8×8 mm.
- A vertical VivaStack can be imaged. It consists of single high-resolution images acquired from the top skin surface up to 200 µm, corresponding to the papillary dermis, to obtain a sort of "optic biopsy."

2 RCM FEATURES OF MELANOMA

- Pagetoid spread [4]: Presence of atypical melanocytes, round or dendritic shaped, arranged as single cells or small nests, scattered within the epidermis (a.k.a. epidermotropism or pagetoid melanocytosis)
- Cytologic atypia: Atypical large and bright melanocytes at the DEJ
- Nonspecific architecture:
  - Absence of a "regular" ringed, clod, or meshwork pattern as usually seen in common nevi
  - Obvious interruption of the architecture with the onset of the so-called nonedged papillae (papillae with ill-defined contour)
- Melanocytes infiltrating dermal papillae and atypical nesting (dense and sparse nests, sheet-like structures, cerebriform nests [5–7])

3 LENTIGO MALIGNA

- Look for:
  - Pagetoid spread, mainly composed of dendritic-shaped melanocytes located around hair follicle [3]
  - Junctional nesting arranged in a medusa-like pattern (Fig. 3.3.1):
    - Confocal structures of LM are listed in Table 3.3.1.
- Differential diagnosis:
  - Pigmented actinic keratosis (overlapping feature: presence of dendritic melanocytes in the epidermis)

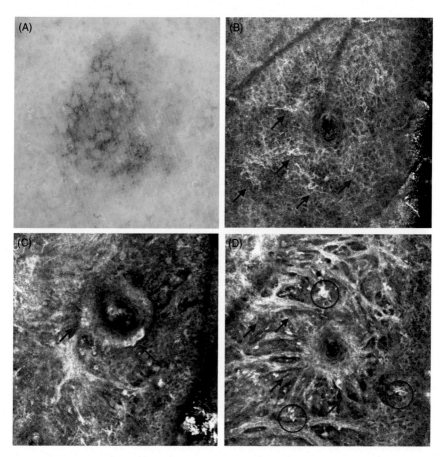

FIGURE 3.3.1   **Lentigo maligna.** (A) Dermoscopy reveals the presence of gray dots arranged to form polygons. (B) RCM shows the presence of pagetoid cells (*arrows*) with dendritic shape located around the hair follicle (*asterisk*). (C) Atypical melanocytes (*arrows*) can be seen along the hair follicle (*asterisk*) at dermoepidermal junctional level. (D) A typical medusa-like pattern with junctional nests (*arrows*) arising from the hair follicle (*asterisk*) can be seen as well as the presence of large atypical melanocytes (*circles*). *RCM*, Reflectance confocal microscopy.

- Diagnostic pearls:
  - Dealing with facial lesions the question is not whether the lesion is benign or malignant but it is rather whether the tumor is melanocytic or not. Thus, the recognition of nesting is mandatory to increase the diagnostic confidence and decide whether to biopsy or not a given lesion.
  - RCM can be used for a presurgical mapping of LM that often may present indistinct clinical borders.

TABLE 3.3.1   RCM Features for Melanoma Diagnosis

Melanoma subtype	Epidermis	DEJ	Dermis
Lentigo maligna	Pagetoid cells with dendritic shape Located around the hair follicle	Nonedged DP Junctional nests (medusa-like pattern)	Melanophages, solar elastosis (curled fibers)
Superficial spreading melanoma	Widespread/focal round/dendritic pagetoid cells	Ringed/meshwork/ nonspecific pattern Irregular, non-/edged DP Irregular melanocytic nests Junctional thickening Mild-marked atypia	Irregular dermal nest (dense, sparse, cerebriform) Sheet-like structures Plump bright cells Pagetoid cells within DP
Nodular melanoma	Thinning of the epidermis Widespread/focal round/dendritic pagetoid cells	Disarrayed DEJ Pleomorphic cells in sheet-like structures Atypical cells	Dermal nests (sheet-like structures, cerebriform) Enlarged blood vessels

DP, Dermal papillae; RCM, reflectance confocal microscopy.

4 SUPERFICIAL SPREADING MELANOMA

- Look for:
  - The presence of focal pagetoid spread or widespread distribution [3–9]
  - Pagetoid cells that display a roundish shape with short and thick dendrites and prominent black nuclei (Fig. 3.3.2)
  - Nonedged contours of the dermal papillae
  - Loss of the papillary dermal contours
  - Infiltration by atypical bright round or dendritic cells
  - Irregularly shaped, discohesive nests in the papillary dermis (Fig. 3.3.3):
    - Confocal structures of SSM are listed in Table 3.3.1 (Fig. 3.3.1).

5 NODULAR MELANOMA

- Look for:
  - Flattened epidermis, with few pagetoid cells [10]

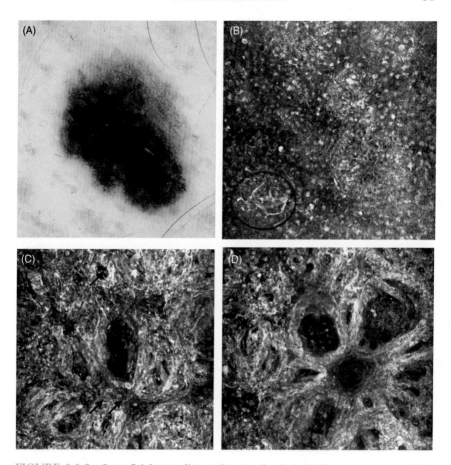

FIGURE 3.3.2 **Superficial spreading melanoma (in situ).** (A) Dermoscopy reveals the presence of atypical pigmented network with different shade of brown color. (B) Pagetoid cells (*circle*) with larger size compared to surrounding keratinocytes can be seen at epidermal level. (C) Cytologic atypia with rounded melanocytes (*arrows*) located around nonedged papillae is present at DEJ level. (D) Architectural disarray with junctional nesting composed of dendritic melanocytes.

- A total filling of the epidermis by an upward migration of melanocyte nests and pagetoid melanocytes as single cells (Fig. 3.3.4)
- Sheet-like structures of large and multinucleated melanocytes at the DEJ
- Cerebriform nests
- Enlarged and tortuous vessels

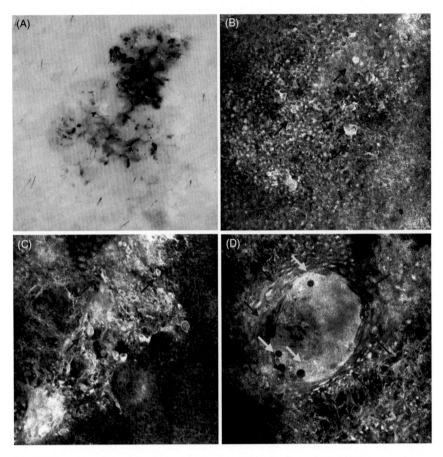

FIGURE 3.3.3 **Superficial spreading melanoma (microinvasive).** (A) Dermoscopy reveals an asymmetric lesion with irregularly distributed brown and black globules and bluish structures. (B) Round-shaped, large pagetoid cells with bright cytoplasm (*arrows*) are observed at epidermal layer. (C) Sheet-like structure with pleomorphic cells (*arrows*) can be seen at dermal level. (D) Moreover, dense and sparse nests (*red arrows*) with atypical melanocytes (*yellow arrows*) are detected.

6 MUCOSAL MELANOMA

- Look for:
  - The presence of roundish cells
  - A high density of dendritic cells with atypia
  - Intraepithelial bright cells

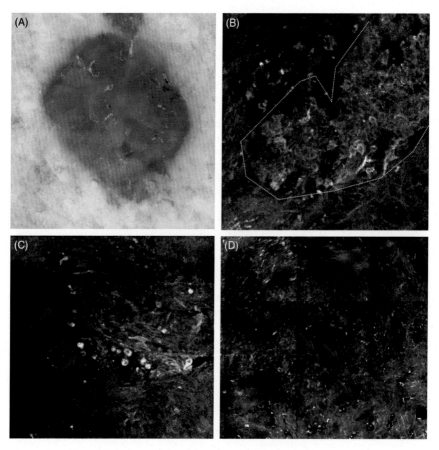

FIGURE 3.3.4 **Nodular melanoma.** (A) Dermoscopically, the tumor is typified by a bluish homogeneous color with few brown dots. (B) Sheet-like nesting (*dashed line*) with malignant melanocytes (*arrows*) is present. (C) Atypical bright melanocytes (*arrows*) located in a vessel as sign of vascular invasion. (D) The presence of cerebriform nests (*arrows*) corresponding to a solid dermal proliferation represents a significant and highly specific clue for melanoma diagnosis.

7 FINAL REMARKS

RCM disclose a new morphologic universe that is close to histopathology with the added value of being performed in vivo and over time. Because of its high sensitivity for detecting melanomas at early stages, RCM reduces the risk of referring a melanoma for monitoring and eventually losing a patient to follow-up. It can also decrease the number of unnecessary biopsies of benign melanocytic lesions.

References

[1] Pellacani G, Cesinaro AM, Seidenari S. Reflectance-mode confocal microscopy of pigmented skin lesions—improvement in melanoma diagnostic specificity. J Am Acad Dermatol 2005;53:979–85.

[2] Pellacani G, Guitera P, Longo C, Avramidis M, Seidenari S, Menzies S. The impact of in vivo reflectance confocal microscopy for the diagnostic accuracy of melanoma and equivocal melanocytic lesions. J Invest Dermatol 2007;127:2759–65.

[3] Guitera P, Pellacani G, Crotty KA, Scolyer RA, Li LX, Bassoli S, et al. The impact of in vivo reflectance confocal microscopy on the diagnostic accuracy of lentigo maligna and equivocal pigmented and nonpigmented macules of the face. J Invest Dermatol 2010;130(8):2080–91.

[4] Pellacani G, Cesinaro AM, Seidenari S. Reflectance-mode confocal microscopy for the in vivo characterization of pagetoid melanocytosis in melanomas and nevi. J Invest Dermatol 2005;125(3):532–7.

[5] Pellacani G, Cesinaro AM, Seidenari S. In vivo confocal reflectance microscopy for the characterization of melanocytic nests and correlation with dermoscopy and histology. Br J Dermatol 2005;152:384–6.

[6] Pellacani G, Longo C, Malvehy J, Puig S, Carrera C, Segura S, et al. In vivo confocal microscopic and histopathologic correlations of dermoscopic features in 202 melanocytic lesions. Arch Dermatol 2008;144(12):1597–608.

[7] Guitera P, Menzies SW, Longo C, Cesinaro AM, Scolyer RA, Pellacani G. In vivo confocal microscopy for diagnosis of melanoma and basal cell carcinoma using a two-step method: analysis of 710 consecutive clinically equivocal cases. J Invest Dermatol 2012;132(10):2386–94.

[8] Guitera P, Moloney FJ, Menzies SW, Stretch JR, Quinn MJ, Hong A, et al. Improving management and patient care in lentigo maligna by mapping with in vivo confocal microscopy. JAMA Dermatol 2013;149(6):692–8.

[9] Pellacani G, De Pace B, Reggiani C, Cesinaro AM, Argenziano G, Zalaudek I, et al. Distinct melanoma types based on reflectance confocal microscopy. Exp Dermatol 2014;23(6):414–8.

[10] Segura S, Pellacani G, Puig S, Longo C, Bassoli S, Guitera P, et al. In vivo microscopic features of nodular melanomas: dermoscopy, confocal microscopy, and histopathologic correlates. Arch Dermatol 2008;144(10):1311–20. [Erratum in Arch Dermatol 2009;145(5):556].

Further Reading

Rajadhyaksha M, Grossman M, Esterowitz D, Webb RH, Anderson RR. In vivo confocal scanning laser microscopy of human skin: melanin provides strong contrast. J Invest Dermatol 1995;104:946–52.

Rajadhyaksha M, Gonzalez S, Zavislan JM, Anderson RR, Web RH. In vivo confocal laser microscopy of human skin II: advances in instrumentation and comparison with histology. J Invest Dermatol 1999;113:293–303.

Pellacani G, Scope A, Ferrari B, Pupelli G, Bassoli S, Longo C, et al. New insights into nevogenesis: in vivo characterization and follow-up of melanocytic nevi by reflectance confocal microscopy. J Am Acad Dermatol 2009;61(6):1001–13.

Pellacani G, Cesinaro AM, Longo C, Grana C, Seidenari S. Microscopic in vivo description of cellular architecture of dermoscopic pigment network in nevi and melanomas. Arch Dermatol 2005;141:147–54.

Longo C, Rito C, Beretti F, Cesinaro AM, Piñeiro-Maceira J, Seidenari S, et al. De novo melanoma and melanoma arising from pre-existing nevus: in vivo morphologic differences as evaluated by confocal microscopy. J Am Acad Dermatol 2011;65(3):604–14.

Longo C, Farnetani F, Moscarella E, de Pace B, Ciardo S, Ponti G, et al. Can noninvasive imaging tools potentially predict the risk of ulceration in invasive melanomas showing blue and black colors? Melanoma Res 2013;23(2):125–31.

Longo C, Farnetani F, Ciardo S, Cesinaro AM, Moscarella E, Ponti G, et al. Is confocal microscopy a valuable tool in diagnosing nodular lesions? A study of 140 cases. Br J Dermatol 2013;169(1):58–67.

Debarbieux S, Perrot JL, Erfan N, Ronger-Savlé S, Labeille B, Cinotti E, et al. Reflectance confocal microscopy of mucosal pigmented macules: a review of 56 cases including 10 macular melanomas. Br J Dermatol 2014;170(6):1276–84.

Pellacani G, Pepe P, Casari A, Longo C. Reflectance confocal microscopy as a second-level examination in skin oncology improves diagnostic accuracy and saves unnecessary excisions: a longitudinal prospective study. Br J Dermatol 2014;171(5):1044–51.

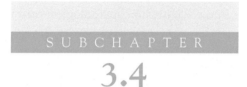

SUBCHAPTER

3.4

The Histopathological Diagnosis

Gerardo Ferrara

Macerata General Hospital, Macerata, Italy

For clinicopathological purposes, it is still useful to refer to the classification proposed by Clark et al. [1] (the United States) and McGovern [2] (Australia) where categories are identified by the microscopic features of the intraepidermal component of the neoplasm. When such an intraepidermal component is not associated with an invasive dermal component (melanoma cells breeching the basal membrane at the dermoepidermal junction), melanoma is defined as "in situ" (confined within its anatomic compartment of origin).

1 CLASSICAL (CLARK'S AND MCGOVERN'S) SUBTYPES OF MELANOMA

1.1 Lentigo Maligna Melanoma

- Look for:
  - Lentiginous (which is mainly a single cell) proliferation, mostly along the basal layer of the epidermis, with deep involvement of the adnexal structures:
    - Proliferation of melanocytes in the depth of the adnexa may mimic invasion [3].

- Spindle neoplastic melanocytes with nuclear pleomorphism
- Severe solar elastosis of the dermis (the histological hallmark of a severe and chronic sun damage)
- Atrophy of the epidermis:
  - Long-standing lesions of lentigo maligna may show a "nested" architecture [4] (nest: an aggregate of at least three melanocytes).
- Differential diagnosis:
  - Subacute/chronic melanocytic photoactivation: Epithelioid and monotonously atypical melanocytes without nesting and pigmentation (the latter being present in a cap-like fashion in the supranuclear region of the nearby keratinocytes) [5]
- Diagnostic pearls:
  - Take always into account clinicopathological correlation.

1.2 Superficial Spreading Melanoma

- Look for:
  - Melanocytes at all levels of the epidermis (pagetoid pattern)
  - Epithelioid neoplastic melanocytes with hyperchromatic nucleus and an abundant pale cytoplasm with "dusty" melanin (pagetoid cells)
- These features impart a "shotgun appearance" to the epidermis.
- Pagetoid configuration is not pathognomonic of melanoma. When pagetoid configuration is made by relatively small cells, it is at risk of being overlooked on histopathological examination.
- Differential diagnosis:
  - Pagetoid scatter may be found in vulvar/genital nevi, acral nevi, recurrent/persistent nevi, Spitz/Reed nevi, in nevi of the childhood, and in several nonmelanocytic tumors (Paget's disease, pagetoid Bowen's disease, tricholemmal carcinoma, epidermotropic T-cell lymphoma, Merkel cell carcinoma, Langerhans cell histiocytosis).
  - Epidermotropic metastasis of melanoma.
- Diagnostic pearls:
  - In favor of a diagnosis of superficial spreading melanoma in the case of a melanocytic tumor: Widespread pagetoid configuration, pagetoid configuration at the edges of the tumor, and cytologic atypia [6]
  - Anamnestic data and clinicopathological correlation

1.3 Nodular Melanoma

- Look for:
  - An intraepidermal neoplastic component that involves less than three rete ridges at the edges of a dermal tumor mass:
    - Some cases fulfilling the criteria for nodular melanoma represent a bona fide advanced nodular phase of another subtype of melanoma [7].

- Also nevoid melanoma and spitzoid melanoma (see the subsequent text) should have, by definition, the typical architectural features of nodular melanoma.
- Differential diagnosis:
  - Metastatic melanoma
- Diagnostic pearls:
  - In favor of primary nodular melanoma is the prominent involvement of the epidermis, the association with a nevus, and the presence of an epidermal "collarette" at the edges of the neoplastic nodule.

1.4 Acral (and Mucosal) Lentiginous Melanoma

- Look for:
  - A lentiginous intraepidermal component with a striking predominance of spindle melanocytes with hyperchromatic nuclei, mainly arranged in single units at the junction
  - Variable (not always prominent) pagetoid spread [8]
  - Hyperplastic epithelium, usually with thin and very elongated rete ridges
  - Collections of lymphocytes at the tips of the rete ridges (inflammation, often evident even in very early lesions) [9]:
    - Tumors showing these features have been described in the volar skin, in the nail matrix, in the oral and nasal cavity, in the vulva, and in the anus [10].

2 OTHER SUBTYPES OF MELANOMA

The WHO 2006 classification of melanoma [11] (Table 3.4.1) encompasses, along with the "classical" subtypes, the following specified entities:

- *Desmoplastic and desmoplastic neurotropic melanoma*:
  - A spindle cell melanoma in which the malignant cells are separated by collagen fibers or fibrous stroma. Lymphoid (lymphofollicular) nodules are a common key feature. Neurotropism (perineural or intraneural growth often extending far from the bulk of the tumor) is seen in at least 30% of cases [11].
  - It typically arises on chronically sun-damaged skin (and in these cases pushes solar elastosis into the deep dermis).
  - The histopathological diagnosis can be very difficult: an atypical junctional component may be scanty or absent, cellularity may be low, and cytologic atypia may be subtle. In addition, desmoplastic melanoma full-blown dermoplasic melanoma

TABLE 3.4.1   Histological Subtypes of Melanoma According to the WHO 2006
Classification [11]

Superficial spreading melanoma (8743/3)

Nodular melanoma (8721/3)

Lentigo maligna (8742/2)

Acral lentiginous melanoma (8744/3)

Desmoplastic and desmoplastic neurotropic melanoma (8745/3)

Melanoma arising from blue nevus (8780/3)

Melanoma arising in a giant congenital nevus (8761/3)

Melanoma of childhood

Nevoid melanoma (8720/3)

Persistent melanoma (8720/3)

In parentheses is the morphology code of the International Classification of Diseases for Oncology
(ICD-O) and the Systematized Nomenclature of Medicine (http://snomed.org).
Behavior is coded /0 for benign tumors, /3 for malignant tumors, /2 for noninvasive tumors, and /1 for
borderline or uncertain behavior.

is negative to the most commonly used panmelanocytic
immunohistochemical markers (positive only to S100, p75/NGFr,
SOX10).
- In order to define a melanoma as "desmoplastic" the above-
  described immunomorphologic features must be present in
  >90% of the tumor mass (desmoplastic features can be focal
  changes in other subtypes of melanoma, as well as in recurrences
  and metastases) [12].

- *Melanoma arising from blue nevus*:
  - Primary dermal melanoma that arises in the context of a dermal
    dendritic cell proliferation (the so-called "blue nevus family" [13]),
    most commonly a cellular blue nevus [14,15]
  - The most common anatomic locations being the same as blue nevi
    (head/neck, trunk, buttock/sacrococcygeum) [14,15]
  - Typically biphasic histopathology: Abrupt transition from the
    benign to the overtly malignant counterpart

- *Melanoma arising in a giant congenital nevus*:
  - A melanoma arising either at the junction or within the dermis
    in the context of a giant (>20 cm in diameter [16]) congenital
    nevus [11].
  - The lifetime risk of melanoma in giant congenital nevi is
    approximately 2%–5%, with most melanomas arising in the first
    decade of life [17,18].

- *Childhood melanoma*:
  - In utero to the birth ("congenital melanoma")
  - From the birth to 1 year of age ("neonatal melanoma")
  - From 1 year of age to puberty ("childhood melanoma," sensu strictiori) [11]
  - Childhood melanoma can be histopathologically subclassified into:
    - Conventional (adult-type)
    - Small cell (resembling a lymphoma or another small round blue cell malignancy)
    - Resembling Spitz nevus [11]: The most controversial category (we personally restrict the term "spitzoid melanoma of the childhood" to cases characterized by an overtly malignant, nonspitzoid melanocytic clone developing in the background of a spitzoid neoplasm) [19,20]

- *Nevoid melanoma*:
  - It is a subtype of nodular melanoma mimicking the architectural features of a common compound or intradermal nevus.
  - Two histopathological variants can be recognized: verrucous (papillated) nodular/plaque-like (nonpapillated)
  - Histopathologically:
    - Confluent growth of melanocytes, often in vertically oriented sheets
    - Minimal or even absent junctional component (especially in the nodular variant)—on the contrary there can be effacement of the epidermis and loss of the subepidermal "grenz zone"
  - Cytomorphologically:
    - "Pseudomaturation" (progressive reduction of the size of the nests and of the cells from the surface to the depth)
    - Pleomorphism and mitotic figures, even in the deep portion of the tumor, being almost invariably seen [21]
  - Immunostain for Ki67 (evidence of irregularly distributed positive cells in clusters and/or within the deep portion of the tumor) can assist the diagnosis [22].

- *Persistent melanoma*:
  - Persistent growth of an incompletely excised primary melanoma. It extends beyond the surgical scar in the same growth pattern as the tumor left on the surgical margin(s) of the previous (excision) specimen. Inflammation and fibrosis are prominent. It must be distinguished from:
  - Recurrent nevus [23]:
    - Recurrency in few months
    - Centered on the scar
    - Typical trizonal pattern (atypical, usually heavily pigmented junctional component/wide area of dermal fibrosis/bland-appearing deep dermal melanocytic component) (Fig. 3.4.2)

- Local (in-transit) metastasis of completely excised melanoma [24]:
  - Recurrency in several years
  - Distance from the scar
  - Multinodular growth pattern
  - Frequent vascular invasion
  - Absence of the host response
- *Other subtypes of melanoma* are not listed in the WHO 2006 classification and are given in Table 3.4.2.

TABLE 3.4.2   Other Histological Variants of Melanoma

"Invisible" (achromic) melanoma	Epitheliomorphic neoplastic cells with no melanin deposition; not uncommon as an in situ neoplasm on chronically sun-damaged skin
Small-diameter melanoma	A melanoma whose breadth is <6 mm in vivo; <4.7 mm after formalin fixation
Nested melanoma of the elderly	Junctional proliferation almost exclusively composed of large and irregular nests
Primary dermal melanoma	Melanocytic tumor in dermis or subcutis with no in situ component (regression of the intraepidermal component or derivation from nonepidermal melanocytes)
Polypoid/exophytic melanoma	Cauliflower-like pattern; cytologic atypia usually striking
Verrucous melanoma	Melanoma with a prominent papillated epidermal hyperplasia
Follicular melanoma	Neoplastic growth centered on one to three hair follicles; length of the epidermal involvement to each side of the affected hair follicle(s) not exceeding the depth of the follicular structure
Minimal deviation melanoma	Possibly a variant of nevoid melanoma, with a minimal histological deviation from a "common" or a "dysplastic" nevus
Small cell melanoma	Small tumor cells, with minimal cytoplasm, round, hyperchromatic nuclei and prominent nucleoli
Signet ring melanoma	Tumor cells with pale cytoplasmic globular inclusions pushing the nucleus at the periphery
Rhabdoid melanoma	Large epithelioid tumor cells showing an abundant inclusion-like eosinophilic cytoplasm
Balloon and clear cell melanoma	Tumor cells with an abundant clear cytoplasm with fine granular or vacuolar change
Myxoid melanoma	Tumor cells interspersed within an intercellular matrix made by a basophilic, PAS-negative and Alcian blue–positive mucinous material

TABLE 3.4.2   Other Histological Variants of Melanoma (*cont.*)

Melanoma with neuroendocrine features	Carcinoid-like pattern; paraganglioma-like pattern; neuroblastic-like pattern. Possible immunohistochemical expression of chromogranin A and synaptophysin, with or without the above-detailed morphologic features
Pseudovascular melanoma	Angiotropic melanoma cells around and infiltrating vessel walls, or angiomatoid changes with blood-filled spaces reminiscent of angiosarcoma
Sarcomatous (spindle cell) melanoma	A spindle cell malignant tumor; often showing loss of some panmelanocytic markers
Pseudolymphomatous melanoma	Melanoma with prominent lymphoid cell infiltrate; melanoma cells with some degree of cohesiveness (lymphoepithelioma-like pattern)
Bullous/acantholytic melanoma	Junctional confluence of discohesive melanocytes creating a bullous cleft
Melanoma with multinucleated giant cells	Touton-like, osteoclast-like, or pleomorphic giant cells interspersed within the tumor mass
Melanoma with monster cells	Tumor cells of gigantic size
Metaplastic melanoma	Melanoma with metaplastic elements such as bone, cartilage, and smooth muscle
BAP-1 mutation associated melanoma	Melanoma cells with somewhat spitzoid cytomorphologic features resulting from biallelic inactivating mutation of the BAP-1 gene on 3p21.1; diagnosis confirmed by a negative nuclear immunostain for the BAP-1 protein in neoplastic cells

3 HISTOPATHOLOGICAL DIAGNOSIS

Optimal evaluation of any melanocytic lesion requires complete excision that incorporates the full thickness of the involved lesion removed intact. Avoid:

- Shave procedures: Do not include the intact base of the lesion.
- Punch procedures: Limitations due to the "sampling" of the lesions. They must be restricted to the preoperative differential diagnosis between melanocytic and nonmelanocytic lesions whose in toto excision would lead to cosmetic and/or functional impairment.

Figs. 3.4.1 and 3.4.2 illustrate the main histopathological features of melanoma. Table 3.4.3 summarizes the main differential criteria between nevus and melanoma.

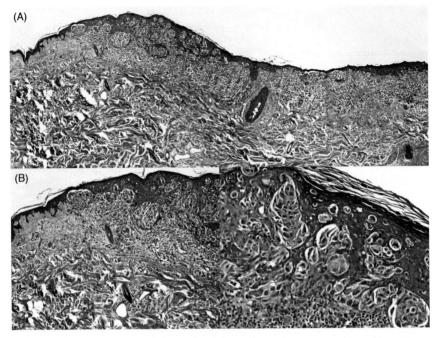

FIGURE 3.4.1 A large, strikingly asymmetric, melanocytic tumor with regression (A), irregular nesting (B), and prominent pagetoid configuration (C).

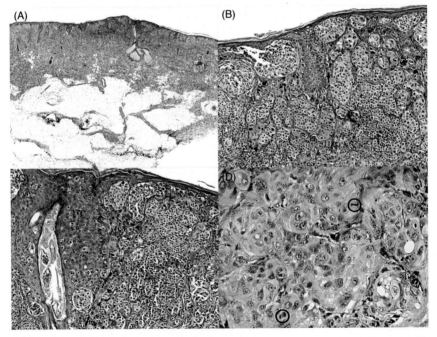

FIGURE 3.4.2 A melanoma of the face characterized by an uneven distribution of the pigmentation (A), different cell types at the same microscopic levels (B), adnexal involvement with pagetoid pattern (C), and striking cytologic atypia (D) with mitotic figures (*circles*).

TABLE 3.4.3 Histopathological Criteria for the Differential Diagnosis Between Nevus and Melanoma

Nevus	Melanoma
Architectural criteria	
Size	
With the exception of congenital nevi, a nevus is seldom larger than 8 mm	A diameter >8 mm is the rule
Symmetry	
Nevi are symmetric: an ideal perpendicular line passing through the center of the lesion divides the tumor into two specularly similar halves	Melanomas are asymmetric
Pigment distribution	
Melanin is uniformly distributed and, with the exception of dermal dendritic melanocytic tumors, mainly confined within the superficial part of benign lesions	Melanin is irregularly distributed; largely amelanotic tumors can show pigment synthesis in the depth
Nests	
Uniformly sized, shaped, and spaced junctional nests prevail over single cells. In Spitz nevus and in "dysplastic" nevus there can be focal junctional fusion ("bridging") of nests	Single cells prevail over nests; the latter are irregularly sized, shaped, and spaced; junctional fusion of nests is irregular
Cytologic criteria	
Cell distribution	
Monotonous cell population; regular spacing of the nuclei; same cell population at the same level of both the epidermis and the dermis	Hypercellularity, crowding/overlapping of nuclei; different cell populations at the same levels of the epidermis and/or of the dermis
Mitoses	
Few and confined within the superficial part of the lesions	Common; superficial and deep; often within the "proliferation belt" (within 0.25 mm from the growing lateral and deep edges of the tumor in the dermis)
Atypia	
Absent; "random" (nonconfluent) in Spitz nevus	Present, confluent
Necrosis	
Absent	Present
Maturation	
Progressive reduction of the cell size with the descent into the dermis: epithelioid (type A) melanocytes at the junction; lymphocyte-like (type B) melanocytes within the superficial dermis; neuroid (type C) melanocytes within the deep dermis	The cell size does not significantly change from the surface to the depth; different cell clones at the same levels; no neuroid melanocytes in the depth

(Continued)

TABLE 3.4.3   Histopathological Criteria for the Differential Diagnosis Between Nevus and Melanoma (*cont.*)

Nevus	Melanoma
Pagetoid configuration	
Absent or confined within the central portion of the lesion	Present, irregularly distributed, also close to the lateral edges of the tumor
Dermoepidermal changes	
Epidermis	
Regular hyperplasia: thin and elongated rete ridges in "dysplastic" nevus; broad rete ridges with overlying hyperkeratosis/hypergranulosis in Spitz nevus	Flattening of the dermoepidermal junction; atrophy; consumption; ulceration. Possible irregular hyperplasia
Clefts	
In Spitz nevus, half-moon shaped, with sharp separation of the junctional nests from the nearby keratinocytes	Irregular clefts; horizontal clefts
Kamino bodies	
In Spitz nevus: large, dull pink, numerous, sometimes pigmented	If present, few in number and small in size
Adnexa	
Terminal hair with "hamartomatous" features; hyperplastic sebaceous glands; folliculocentric growth	Terminal hair absent; adnexotropic growth
Elastic fibers	
Hyperplastic; slight or no sun damage	Elastic fibers destroyed; marked sun damage
Inflammation	
Patchy, perivascular. In nevus of Sutton, a broad and symmetric band of lymphocytes involving the entire length of the lesion	Lichenoid, asymmetric. Associated with regression (fibrosis, melanosis, newly formed vessels)

4 IMMUNOHISTOCHEMISTRY

Because of the lack of objective and reproducible diagnostic criteria, ancillary techniques have been increasingly implemented in routine practice. Among these, immunohistochemistry is the most widely used. It is aimed at:

- The demonstration of a melanocytic histogenesis for undifferentiated (anaplastic) malignancies in their either primary cutaneous or metastatic site, comprising the sentinel node:
  - Achieved with the use of "panmelanocytic markers": The best approach is to use S100 (the most sensitive and less expensive

marker) plus one more specific lineage-specific marker (MelanA/ MART1, tyrosinase, MITF1, p75/NGFr, or SOX10).
- In our opinion, the most efficient and less expensive couple of reagents are S100 and MelanA/MART1:
  - Desmoplastic melanoma is consistently negative to lineage-specific markers (useful with the anti-p73/nerve growth factor receptor antibody, or with the anti-SOX10 antibody) [25].
- The identification of tricky malignancies:
  - On sun-damaged skin, a nuclear marker (MITF1 or SOX10) should replace MelanA/MART1, as "pseudomelanocytic nests" of keratinocytes involved in a lichenoid tissue reaction can be labeled [26].
- The identification of prognostic factors (comprising Breslow's thickness) in melanoma:
  - Stain of deeply entrapped melanocytes thereby avoiding undermicrostaging (cases of melanoma with halo reaction and/or regression with "blurred" deep margins) [27]
  - Identification of mitotic figures by immunodetection of phosphohistone H3 protein [28]
- The differential diagnosis among benign and malignant melanocytic tumors in the skin (the most ambitious task for immunohistochemistry):
  - An acceptable compromise between cost, effectiveness, and increase in technical routine workload is the adoption of an antibody panel composed as follows:
    - The anti–cell cycle–related protein Ki67. Its staining can be evaluated either with a systematic count of neoplastic cells (<5% of neoplastic cells labeled in common nevi; 5%–13% of neoplastic cells labeled in "dysplastic" nevi and Spitz nevi; >13% of neoplastic cells labeled in melanoma) or with an "eyeballed" evaluation of the staining pattern (tidy in nevi; untidy with clusters of proliferating cells in melanoma) [22,29].
    - The anti–human melanoma black 45 (HMB45) [30]. Its expression recalls the "maturation" of nevi (progressive loss of reactivity from the surface to the depth) and the architectural disorder of melanoma ("patchy" reactivity, with isolated or clustered cells being labeled throughout the dermis) [22,30].
    - The anti-p16 protein. This antibody stains nevi in either a strong and diffuse or a tidy ("checkerboard") pattern; instead, melanomas typically show confluent foci of complete loss of reactivity [30,31].
      - Unfortunately, the above-illustrated rules have relevant exceptions and limitations (e.g., in melanoma progression the HMB45+ is lost [32]; benign dermal dendritic melanocytic

proliferations are HMB45+ and a focal loss of reactivity can be a clue to malignancy [22]).

- Immunohistochemistry must be always evaluated within the morphologic context, and not any single immunostain is able to give clear-cut information for the differential diagnosis between nevus and melanoma.

5 HISTOPATHOLOGICAL REPORTING OF MELANOMA

The histopathological report must include all the pertinent clinical information and a thorough macroscopic description comprising the sampling protocol adopted. A microscopic description of the tumor is optional if the final diagnosis is clear-cut.

Compulsory histopathological parameters include the following:

- Ulceration (present vs. absent):
  - A full-thickness epidermal defect above dermal melanoma growth, with reactive tissue changes (fibrin, neutrophils) and atrophy or hypertrophy of the surrounding epidermis, with no history of trauma or surgery [33]
- Regression (if present):
  - Replacement of a portion of dermal tumor tissue by fibrosis with newly formed vessels and a variable amount of lymphocytes and melanophages. It can be the following:
    - Focal (involving a portion of invasive tumor)
    - Partial (involving the entire invasive tumor)
    - Complete (involving the entire tumor)
  - Since complete regression and regression involving more than 75% of the lesion carry adverse prognostic importance in invasive melanoma [34], it is recommended to assess regression, if present, as follows:
    - Involving up to 75% of the tumor mass
    - Involving more than 75% of the tumor mass
    - Involving the entire tumor (complete)
- Lymphovascular invasion (if present):
  - The immunostain for an endothelial marker (CD31, podoplanin) can help the assessment [35].
- Perineural invasion (if present):
  - Melanoma and nerves are S100-positive. An immunostain for the perineural sheath with the anti–epithelial membrane antigen (EMA) or, else, with the anti-Glut1 antibodies can be used to individuate the nerve fibers.

- Breslow's thickness:
  - Maximum tumor thickness is measured with a calibrated ocular micrometer at a right angle to the overlying normal skin.
  - The upper point of reference is the granular layer of the epidermis of the overlying skin or, if the lesion is ulcerated, the base of the ulcer.
  - The lower point is the deepest point of tumor invasion (i.e., the leading edge of a single mass or an isolated group of cells deep to the main mass):
    - If the tumor is transected by the deep margin of the specimen, the depth may be indicated as "at least __ mm" with a comment explaining the limitation of thickness assessment. Special problems in the measurement of Breslow's thickness are illustrated in Table 3.4.4.
    - According to the AJCC8 staging system, tumor thichness should be recorded to the nearest 0.1 mm (e.g., melanomas measured as being into the range of 0.75 and 0.84 mm are reported as 0.8 mm in thickness) [35a].
- Microsatellitosis (if present):
  - Tumor nests greater than 0.05 mm in diameter, in the reticular dermis, panniculus, or vessels beneath the principal invasive tumor but separated from it by at least 0.3 mm of normal tissue on the section in which the Breslow measurement was taken [36]. It is also recommended to include microsatellites into Breslow's thickness itself.

TABLE 3.4.4   Problems in the Measurement of Breslow's Thickness

Melanoma subtype	Suggested strategy
Nevus-associated melanoma	Perform immunohistochemistry (anti-Ki67, anti-HMB45, anti-p16); if still in doubt, report the greatest value of thickness with a statement about a possible overestimation due to the (possible) association with a nevus
Verrucous melanoma	Pick a point halfway between the base and the apex of a papillation and measure from there to the deepest melanoma cells
Follicular melanoma	Draw an ideal vertical line passing through the center of the hair follicle and measure the thickest half of the tumor perpendicular to this line
Bullous/acantholytic melanoma	Detract the thickness of the bullous detachment from the total thickness

HMB, Human melanoma black.

- Status of the surgical margins:
  - Microscopically measured distances between tumor and labeled lateral or deep margins:
    - If a lateral margin is involved by tumor, it should be stated whether the tumor is in situ or invasive.

Optional parameters of the histopathological report are the following:

- Histological subtype
- Clark level, which is defined as follows:
  - I: Intraepidermal tumor only
  - II: Tumor present in but does not fill and expand papillary dermis
  - III: Tumor fills and expands papillary dermis
  - IV: Tumor invades reticular dermis
  - V: Tumor invades subcutis [37].
- Tumor growth phase, radial (horizontal) versus vertical
- Tumor-infiltrating lymphocytes (TILs):
  - *Not identified*
  - *Nonbrisk*: Lymphocytes infiltrate melanoma only focally or not along >90% of the base of the vertical growth phase
  - *Brisk*: Lymphocytes diffusely infiltrate >90% of the base of the vertical growth phase:
    - A paucity of TILs is an adverse prognostic factor for cutaneous melanoma [34]. To qualify as TILs, lymphocytes need to surround and disrupt tumor cells of the vertical growth phase.

No longer used in the American Joint Committee on Cancer (AJCC) 8 staging system for subclassifying pT1 tumors

- Mitotic rate:
  - After finding the areas of the dermis containing most mitotic figures, the count is extended to adjacent fields up to covering an area corresponding to 1 mmq (4 microscopic fields at a 400× magnification)—"hot spot" method.
  - The mitotic rate should be given as an integer number; if no mitotic figure is found in the invasive component of the tumor, the mitotic rate must be given as 0 mmq^{-1}.

6 CONCLUSIONS

The proper diagnosis and classification of melanoma is still a great challenge in modern dermatopathology. Most of the currently used parameters were delivered in the late 1960s; molecular techniques are expected to completely change our landscape of histopathology of melanoma within the next few years.

References

[1] Clark WH Jr, From L, Bernardino EA, Mihm MC. The histogenesis and biologic behaviour of primary human malignant melanoma of the skin. Cancer Res 1969;29:705–27.

[2] McGovern VJ. The classification of melanoma and its relationship with prognosis. Pathology 1970;2:85–98.

[3] Tsakok T, Sheth N, Robson A, Gleeson C, Mallipeddi R. Lentigo maligna mimicking invasive melanoma in Mohs surgery: a case report, <http://f1000research.com/articles/3-25/v1> [accessed Nov 8, 2018].

[4] Clark WH Jr, Mihm MH Jr. Lentigo maligna and lentigo maligna melanoma. Am J Pathol 1969;55:39–67.

[5] Hendi A, Broadland DG, Zitelli JA. Melanocytes in long-standing sun-exposed skin. Quantitative analysis using the MART-1 immunostain. Arch Dermatol 2006;142:871–6.

[6] Petronic-Rosic V, Shea CR, Krausz T. Pagetoid melanocytosis: when is it significant? Pathology 2004;36:435–44.

[7] Zalaudek I, Marghoob AA, Scope A, Leinweber B, Ferrara G, Hofmann-Wellenhof R, et al. Three roots to melanoma. Arch Dermatol 2008;144:1375–9.

[8] Arrington JH III, Reed RJ, Ichinose H, Krementz ET. Plantar lentiginous melanoma. A distinctive variant of human cutaneous malignant melanoma. Am J Surg Pathol 1977;1:131–43.

[9] Kim JY, Choi M, Jo SJ, Min HS, Cho KH. Acral lentiginous melanoma: indolent subtype with long radial growth phase. Am J Dermatopathol 2014;36:142–7.

[10] Skin S Rosai J.. Tumors and tumor-like conditions. In: Rosai J, editor. Rosai and Ackerman's surgical pathology. 10th ed. Edinburgh: Elsevier; 2011. p. 160–71.

[11] de Vries E, Bray F, Coebergh GW, Cerroni L, Ruiter DJ, Elder DE, et al. Malignant melanoma: introduction. In: Le Boit PE, Burg G, Weedon D, Sarasin A, editors. World Health Organization classification of tumours—pathology and genetics of skin tumours. Lyon: IARC Press; 2006. p. 52–65.

[12] Busam KJ. Desmoplastic melanoma. Clin Lab Med 2011;31:321–30.

[13] Ferrara G, Soyer HP, Malvehy J, Piccolo D, Puig S, Sopena J, et al. The many faces of blue nevus: a clinicopathologic study. J Cutan Pathol 2007;34:543–51.

[14] Granter SR, McKee PH, Calonje E, Mihm MC Jr, Busam K. Melanoma associated with blue nevus and melanoma mimicking cellular blue nevus: a clinicopathologic study of 10 cases on the spectrum of so-called 'malignant blue nevus'. Am J Surg Pathol 2001;25:316–23.

[15] Loghavi S, Curry JL, Torres-Cabala CA, Ivan D, Patel KP, Mehrotra M, et al. Melanoma arising in association with blue nevus: a clinical and pathologic study of 24 cases and comprehensive review of the literature. Mod Pathol 2014;27:1468–78.

[16] Ruiz-Maldonado R. Measuring congenital melanocytic nevi. Pediatr Dermatol 2004;21:178–9.

[17] Warner C, Dinulos JG. Core concepts in congenital melanocytic nevi and infantile hemangiomas. Curr Opin Pediatr 2014;26:130–5.

[18] Vourc'h-Jourdain M, Martin L, Barbarot S. aRED. Large congenital melanocytic nevi: therapeutic management and melanoma risk: a systematic review. J Am Acad Dermatol 2013;68:493–8.

[19] Ferrara G, Gianotti R, Cavicchini S, Salviato T, Zalaudek I, Argenziano G. Spitz nevus, Spitz tumor and spitzoid melanoma: a comprehensive clinicopathologic overview. Dermatol Clin 2013;31(4):589–98. viii.

[20] Ferrara G, Cavicchini S, Corradin MT. Hypopigmented atypical spitzoid neoplasms (atypical Spitz nevi, atypical Spitz tumors, spitzoid melanoma): a clinicopathological update. Dermatol Pract Concept 2015;5:45–52.

[21] McNutt NS. 'Triggered trap': nevoid malignant melanoma. Semin Diagn Pathol 1998;15:203–9.

[22] Prieto VG, Shea CR. Immunohistochemistry of melanocytic proliferations. Arch Pathol Lab Med 2011;135:853–9.

[23] Fox JC, Reed JA, Shea CR. The recurrent nevus phenomenon: a history of challenge, controversy, and discovery. Arch Pathol Lab Med 2011;135:842–6.

[24] Ferrara G, Zalaudek I. Is histopathological overdiagnosis of melanoma a good insurance for the future? Melanoma Manag 2015;2:21–5.

[25] Weissinger SE, Keil P, Silvers DN, Klaus BM, Möller P, Horst BA, et al. A diagnostic algorithm to distinguish desmoplastic from spindle cell melanoma. Mod Pathol 2014;27:524–34.

[26] Beltraminelli H, Shabrawi-Caelen LE, Kerl H, Cerroni L. Melan-a positive 'pseudomelanocytic nests': a pitfall in the histopathologic and immunohistochemical diagnosis of pigmented lesions on sun-damaged skin. Am J Dermatopathol 2009;31:305–8.

[27] Drabeni M, Lopez-Vilaró L, Barranco C, Trevisan G, Gallardo F, Pujol RM. Differences in tumor thickness between hematoxylin and eosin and melan-A immunohistochemically stained primary cutaneous melanomas. Am J Dermatopathol 2013;135:56–63.

[28] Tetzlaff MT, Curry JL, Ivan D, Wang WL, Torres-Cabala CA, Bassett RL, et al. Immunodetection of phosphohistone H3 as a surrogate of mitotic figure count and clinical outcome in cutaneous melanoma. Mod Pathol 2013;26:1153–60.

[29] Wasserman J, Maddox J, Racz M, Petronic-Rosic V. Update on immunohistochemical methods relevant to dermatopathology. Arch Pathol Lab Med 2009;133:1053–61.

[30] Ohsie SJ, Sarantopoulos P, Cochran AJ, Binder SW. Immunohistochemical characteristics of melanoma. J Cutan Pathol 2008;35:433–44.

[31] George E, Polissar NL, Wick M. Immunohistochemical evaluation of 16INK4A, e-cadherin, and cyclin D1 expression in melanoma and Spitz tumors. Am J Clin Pathol 2010;133:370–9.

[32] Orchard GE. Comparison of the immunohistochemical labelling of melanocyte differentiation antibodies melan-A, tyrosinase and HMB45 with NKIC3 and S100 protein in the evaluation of benign nevi and malignant melanoma. Histochem J 2000;32:475–81.

[33] Batistatou A, Gököz O, Cook MG, Massi D. Dermatopathology Working Group of the European Society of Pathology. Melanoma histopathology report: proposal for a standardized terminology. Virchows Arch 2011;458:359–61.

[34] Crowson AN, Magro CM, Mihm MC. Prognosticators of melanoma, the melanoma report, and the sentinel lymph node. Mod Pathol 2006;19(Suppl. 2):S71–87.

[35] Aung PP, Leone D, Feller JK, Yang S, Hernandez M, Yaar R, et al. Microvessel density, lymphovascular density, and lymphovascular invasion in primary cutaneous melanoma—correlation with histopathologic prognosticators and BRAF status. Hum Pathol 2015;46:304–12.

[35a] Amin MB, Edge S, Greene F, Byrd DR, Brookland RK, Washington MK, Gershenwald JE, Compton CC, Hess KR, Sullivan DC, Jessup JM, Brierley JD, Gaspar LE, Schilsky RL, Balch CM, Winchester DP, Asare EA, Madera M, Gress DM, Meyer LR, editor. AJCC Cancer Staging Manual, 8th ed. New York: Springer; 2017. p. 563–585.

[36] Harrist TJ, Rigel DS, Day CL, et al. "Microscopic satellites" are more highly associated with regional lymph node metastases than is primary melanoma thickness. Cancer 1984;53:2183–7.

[37] American Joint Committee on Cancer. Melanoma of the skin. In: Edge S, Byrd DR, Compton CC, Fritz AG, Greene FL, Trotti A, editors. AJCC cancer staging manual. 7th ed. Berlin: Springer; 2010. p. 325–44.

Further Reading

Ferrara G, Senetta R, Paglierani M, Massi D. Main clues in the pathological diagnosis of melanoma: is molecular genetics helping? Dermatol Ther 2012;25:423–31.

Farrahi F, Egbert BM, Swetter SM. Histologic similarities between lentigo maligna and dysplastic nevus: importance of clinicopathologic distinction. J Cutan Pathol 2005;32:405–12.

Zalaudek I, Cota C, Ferrara G, Moscarella E, Guitera P, Longo C, et al. Flat pigmented macules on sun-damaged skin of the head/neck: junctional nevus, atypical lentiginous nevus, or melanoma in situ? Clin Dermatol 2014;32:88–93.

Ferrara G, Zalaudek I, Argenziano G. Lentiginous melanoma: a distinctive clinicopathological entity. Histopathology 2008;52:523–5.

Heenan PJ, Clay CD. Epidermotropic metastatic melanoma simulating multiple primary melanomas. Am J Dermatopathol 1991;13:396–402.

Cabral R, Brinca A, Cardoso JC, Tellechea O. Nodular malignant melanoma. Or maybe not? Clin Exp Dermatol 2014;39:416–7.

Jaimes N, Chen L, Dusza SW, Carrera C, Puig S, Thomas L, et al. Clinical and dermoscopic characteristics of desmoplastic melanoma. JAMA Dermatol 2013;149:413–21.

Phadke PA, Rakheja D, Le LP, Selim MA, Kapur P, Davis A, et al. Proliferative nodules arising within congenital melanocytic nevi: a histologic, immunohistochemical, and molecular analysis of 43 cases. Am J Surg Pathol 2011;35:656–69.

Zayour M, Lazova R. Congenital melanocytic nevi. Clin Lab Med 2011;31:267–80.

Neuhold JC, Friesenhahn J, Gerdes N, Krengel S. Case reports of fatal or metastasizing melanoma in children and adolescents: a systematic review of the literature. Pediatr Dermatol 2015;32:13–22.

Cerroni L, Barnhill R, Elder D, Gottlieb G, Heenan P, Kutzner H, et al. Melanocytic tumors of uncertain malignant potential: results of a tutorial held at the XXIX symposium of the International Society of Dermatopathology in Graz, October 2008. Am J Surg Pathol 2010;34:314–26.

Schmoeckel C, Castro CE, Braun-Falco O. Nevoid malignant melanoma. Arch Dermatol Res 1985;277:362–9.

Urso C. A new perspective for Spitz tumors? Am J Dermatopathol 2005;27:364–7.

Ferrara G, Argenziano G, Soyer HP, Corona R, Sera F, Brunetti B, et al. Dermoscopic and histopathologic diagnosis of equivocal melanocytic skin lesions. An interdisciplinary study on 107 cases. Cancer 2002;95:1094–100.

Lefevre M, Vergier B, Balme B, Thiebault R, Delaunay M, Thomas L, et al. Relevance of vertical growth pattern in thin level II cutaneous superficial spreading melanomas. Am J Surg Pathol 2003;27:717–24.

Melanoma Staging

Stefania Borsari*, Caterina Longo**

*Arcispedale Santa Maria Nuova—IRCCS, Reggio Emilia, Italy
**University of Modena and Reggio Emilia, Reggio Emilia, Italy

1 WHAT IS STAGING?

- The word "staging" defines the process of determining how much cancer is in a patient's body and where it is located.
- It allows assigning a number from I to IV, where I refers to localized cancer and IV corresponds to a cancer that has metastasized.
- The stage is based on the results of physical exams, biopsies, and imaging tests (ultrasound, CT or MRI scan) or other tests that have been done.
- Melanoma stage is very important in planning the treatment and estimating the patient's prognosis.

The system most often used to stage melanoma is the American Joint Committee on Cancer (AJCC) TNM system, where:

- *T* stands for *tumor* (how far it has grown within the skin and other factors). The T category is assigned a number (from 0 to 4) based on

Cutaneous Melanoma. http://dx.doi.org/10.1016/B978-0-12-804000-3.00004-1

the tumor's thickness. It may also be assigned a small letter "a" or "b" based on ulceration, as explained in the subsequent text.

- *N* stands for spread to nearby lymph *nodes*. The N category is assigned a number (from 0 to 3) based on whether the melanoma cells have spread to lymph nodes or are found in the lymphatic channels connecting the lymph nodes.
- The *M* category is based on whether the melanoma has *metastasized* (spread) to distant organs, and which organs it has reached.

Cancer staging can be divided into a clinical stage and a pathologic stage that should complement each other: the former is based on all information obtained before the surgical removal of the tumor (by physical and radiologic examinations); the latter adds important information gained by microscopic examination of the tumor by a pathologist.

2 CURRENT STAGING SYSTEM

- The AJCC staging system includes a clinical and a pathologic staging, both outlining five stages (Table 4.1):
  - *0*: in situ disease
  - *I* and *II*: localized disease
    The finding of ulceration in the primary tumor allows differentiating stage I or II "a" from "b" and "c."
  - *III*: regional disease
    This stage can include clinically occult or clinically detected metastases in regional lymph nodes, as well as "in transit metastases" and "satellites."
    The term "regional lymph nodes" refers to lymph node basin that drains lymph from the region around the tumor (e.g., axillary lymph nodes drain lymph from skin of the upper arm).
    - Clinically occult metastases are diagnosed histologically after sentinel lymph node (SLN) biopsy and regional lymph node dissection, when performed.
    - Clinically detected metastases are defined as clinically detectable nodal metastases confirmed by therapeutic lymphadenectomy.
    - In transit metastases are skin or subcutaneous metastases located more than 2 cm from the primary tumor, but are not beyond the regional nodal basin.
    - Satellite lesions are skin or subcutaneous lesions within 2 cm from the primary tumor.

TABLE 4.1   Pathologic Staging for Cutaneous Melanoma According to American Joint Cancer Committee Clinical Staging System [1]

Stage *0*	In situ MM
Stage *IA*	MM < 0.8 mm without ulceration (T1a)
Stage *IB*	0.8–1 mm MM regardless of ulceration or ulcerated MM < 0.8 mm (T1b) MM 1–2 mm without ulceration
Stage *IIA*	MM 1–2 mm with ulceration MM 2–4 mm without ulceration
Stage *IIB*	MM 2–4 mm with ulceration MM > 4 mm without ulceration
Stage *IIC*	MM > 4 mm with ulceration
Stage *IIIA*	MM < 1 mm regardless of ulceration or MM 1–2 mm without ulceration *and* one to three clinically occult metastases in regional lymph nodes
Stage *IIIB*	No evidence of primary tumor *and* one clinically detected metastases in regional lymph nodes or presence of in transit, satellite, and/or microsatellite metastases MM < 1 mm regardless of ulceration or MM 1–2 mm without ulceration *and* one to three metastases in regional lymph nodes, at least one of which clinically detected, or in transit, satellite, and/or microsatellite metastases MM 1–2 mm with ulceration or MM 2–4 mm without ulceration *and* one to three occult or clinically detected metastases in regional lymph nodes or in transit, satellite, and/or microsatellite metastases
Stage *IIIC*	No evidence of primary tumor *and* two or more nodal metastases, at least one of which clinically detected, or in transit, satellite, and/or microsatellite metastases with at least one tumor-involved node or any number of matted nodes with/without in transit, satellite, and/or microsatellite metastases MM < 2 mm regardless of ulceration or MM 2–4 mm without ulceration *and* four or more tumor-involved nodes or in transit, satellite, and/or microsatellite metastases with at least one tumor-involved node or any number of matted nodes with/without in transit, satellite, and/or microsatellite metastases MM 2–4 mm with ulceration or MM > 4 mm without ulceration *and* any metastases in regional lymph nodes and/or presence of in transit, satellite, and/or microsatellite metastases MM > 4 mm with ulceration *and* one to three occult or clinically detected metastases in regional lymph nodes or in transit, satellite, and/or microsatellite metastases with no or one tumor-involved node
Stage *IIID*	MM > 4 mm with ulceration *and* four or more tumor-involved nodes or in transit, satellite, and/or microsatellite metastases with two or more tumor-involved nodes or any number of matted nodes with/without in transit, satellite, and/or microsatellite metastases
Stage *IV*	Any primary MM with any regional lymph node status and distant metastases (to distant skin, subcutis or lymph nodes, or visceral sites)

MM, Melanoma.

■ Despite this distinction, the tumor biology associated with satellite and in transit metastases is similar, so they will have similar treatment or prognosis.

● *IV*: distant metastatic disease

Metastases to lung or other organs (brain, liver, kidneys, adrenal glands, etc.) as well as to distant skin, subcutis, and lymph nodes lead to stage IV.

Clinical staging includes microstaging of the primary melanoma and clinical/radiologic evaluation for metastases. By convention, it should be used after complete excision of the primary melanoma with clinical assessment for regional and distant metastases.

Pathologic staging includes microstaging of the primary melanoma and pathologic information about the regional lymph nodes after partial or complete lymphadenectomy.

3 STAGING PROCEDURE (Fig. 4.1)

1. *Biopsy of primary cutaneous melanoma*:
   a. Perform an excisional biopsy of a suspicious lesion, when possible.
   b. Incisional biopsy for diagnostic purpose is allowed in case of large lesions or lesions located on anatomic areas such as palm/soles and face; there is no evidence that incision of a primary melanoma affects survival or prognosis.
   c. The pathologist will report on the Breslow thickness (corresponding to depth of the melanoma within the skin level measured from stratum granulosum), presence or absence of microscopic ulceration, and mitoses per square millimeter. The pathology report can then be used to assign a preliminary AJCC stage (*0, IA, IB, IIA, IIB,* or *IIC*).
      – In case of *stage 0* melanoma, no further staging procedures should be offered.
      – In case of stage *IA* melanoma, staging will be completed by clinical examination.
      – In cases of *stage IB–IIC* melanoma, it is recommended to proceed with evaluation for regional metastasis that might correspond, in these stages, to SLN biopsy.
2. *Evaluation for regional metastasis*:
   a. Careful palpation of lymph nodes closer to the primary tumor and of the regional area of the primary melanoma: If palpable lymph nodes or dermal/subcutaneous nodules are detected, a fine-needle aspiration or an excision may be performed to obtain a histologic diagnosis.

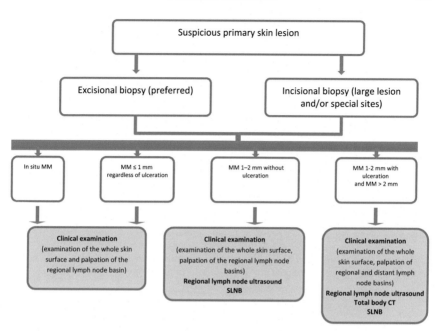

FIGURE 4.1   **Flow chart explaining how to perform staging based on histologic features of the primary cutaneous melanoma.** *MM,* Melanoma; *SLNB,* sentinel lymph node biopsy.

b. In case of invasive melanoma, particularly in case of stage II, lymph node ultrasound is recommended before performing SLN biopsy in order to detect small, nonpalpable, nodal metastasis.

c. If clinical examination (and ultrasound) is negative, proceed with *SLN biopsy*:

– It should be performed at the same time (or before) wide local excision of the primary melanoma.

– Provide the patient detailed verbal and written information about the possible advantages and disadvantages (Table 4.2).

– Contraindications for SLN biopsy are as follows: poor general health status, severe concurrent disease, and poor patient compliance; widespread metastasis (systemic spread of the disease or clinically or sonographically apparent lymph node metastases); and prior wide local excision (since the lymphatic flow from the primary tumor site may be changed).

SLN biopsy is a staging procedure and not therapeutic: this is a crucial point to balance the pros and cons when performing or offering the possibility of SLN to a patient with melanoma. In case of positive SLNB, regional lymph node dissection is usually recommended, at least for those SLN with tumor burden of >1 mm.

TABLE 4.2 Possible Advantages and Disadvantages of Sentinel Lymph Node Biopsy [2]

Advantages	Disadvantages
The technique helps identify whether the cancer has spread to the lymph nodes. It is better than ultrasounds at finding very small nodal metastases	The purpose of the technique is not to cure the cancer. There is no evidence that patients who have SLNB live longer than people who do not have SLNB
The technique can help predict what might happen in the future. For example, in people with a primary MM between 1 and 4 mm: • Around 1 out of 10 die within 10 years if SLNB is negative • Around 3 out of 10 die within 10 years if SLNB is positive	The result needs to be interpreted with caution. Out of 100 people who have a negative SLNB, around 3 will develop a recurrence in the same group of lymph nodes
People who had SLNB could be enrolled in clinical trials of new treatments for MM	A general anesthetic is needed for the surgical procedure
	Complications (e.g., lymphedema, seroma, allergic reaction to radiocolloid) occur in 4%–10% of cases

MM, Melanoma; SLNB, sentinel lymph node biopsy.

3. *Evaluation for distant metastasis*:
   a. The decision to perform a staging procedure should take into account several aspects: the chance to find occult metastases, the chance of false-positive findings, the cost of imaging methods, and whether the findings will lead to a different management.
   b. Early stage melanoma is a cancer with a low incidence of clinically occult disease.
   c. In *asymptomatic patients* with localized cutaneous melanoma of any thickness, baseline blood tests and routine imaging examinations are generally not recommended, since they rarely allow identifying occult systemic disease: they should only be performed as clinically indicated for suspicious signs and symptoms. In addition, currently available treatments for patients with asymptomatic stage IV disease are not associated with better outcomes than intervention when metastases become clinically symptomatic.
      – In case of *stage IA* melanoma, perform only clinical examination (careful observation of the whole skin surface of the patient in order to rule out cutaneous/subcutaneous metastases and palpation of the nodal region closer to the primary tumor).
      – In cases of *stage IB* melanoma, in addition to clinical examination, an ultrasound scan of regional lymph nodes can be offered prior to performing SLN biopsy.

- In case of *stage II* melanoma, clinical examination should include palpation of both regional and distant lymph node basins. An ultrasound scan of regional lymph nodes and a total-body CT scan (brain, neck, thorax, and abdomen) should be performed before performing SLN biopsy.
- Offer total-body CT scan to patients with *stage III* or *suspected stage IV* melanoma.

4 LIMITATIONS OF THE AJCC STAGING SYSTEM

- The AJCC cutaneous melanoma staging system does not always reliably predict patient outcomes by stage and improvements of patient's stratification are still needed.
- For example, patients with a stage IIC melanoma have a worse 5-year overall survival (53%) compared with those who have stage IIIA melanomas (78%). Similarly, 15% of patients with stage I melanoma, which is usually related to an excellent prognosis, could die from melanoma.
- The current understanding of genetic mutations, expression alterations, and host response in cutaneous melanoma probably will lead to new prognostic tools such as molecular and immunologic biomarkers. It has been hypothesized that adding measurements of host antitumor immune response and/or molecular features to staging may improve primary melanoma patients' stratification.

5 TOPIC QUESTIONS

- In which cases is an F-18 fluorodeoxy-D-glucose-positron emission tomography (*FDG-PET*) scan indicated?
  Routine FDG-PET scanning is not recommended for the initial staging evaluation in melanoma patients. A total-body FDG-PET is indicated to confirm suspected visceral metastases visualized by CT scan or ultrasounds. It may also be useful in case of SLN biopsy of head/neck area and in case of stage III melanoma.
- Is there an *age limit* for the SLN biopsy?
  The main benefits from SLN biopsy are regional control and staging information. Staging information can be critical for adjuvant therapy decisions, but the present options for adjuvant therapy in melanoma are poorly tolerated in the *elderly* population and they often are not candidates for clinical trials. In addition, elderly patients have a lower rate of regional involvement, a higher incidence of systemic metastases, and a higher mortality than their younger counterparts.

In patients older than 75 with melanoma 1 mm or thicker, a careful balance regarding the risks and benefits of SLN biopsy should be considered case by case.

Children and young adults with melanoma are more likely to have SLN metastasis and survival analyses indicate that a positive SLN biopsy is a poor prognostic factor in these patients. SLN biopsy is recommended in children and young adults who have a melanoma 1 mm or thicker or with adverse histologic features.

- Is there a benefit to *SLN biopsy* in patients with melanoma thickness >4 mm?

  Clinically lymph node–negative patients with primary tumor thickness >4 mm should be strongly considered for SLN biopsy since SLN status is the most significant prognostic factor among these patients.

- How should patients with *metastases and unknown primary site* be staged?

  When patients have an initial presentation of metastases in the lymph nodes or in the skin or subcutaneous tissues, these should be presumed to be regional (stage III) if an appropriate staging workup does not reveal any other sites of metastases. All other presentations (metastases to visceral sites) should be categorized as stage IV melanoma.

References

[1] American Joint Committee on Cancer (AJCC). Cancer Staging Manual. 8th ed., 2017.
[2] Balch CM, Cascinelli N. Sentinel-node biopsy in melanoma. N Engl J Med 2007; 355(13):1370–1.

Further Reading

Aloia TA, Gershenwald JE, Andtbacka RH, et al. Utility of computer tomography and magnetic resonance imaging staging before completion lymphadenectomy in patients with sentinel lymph node-positive melanoma. J Clin Oncol 2006;24(18):2858–65.
American Joint Committee on Cancer (AJCC). Cancer staging manual. 8th ed. New York: Springer; 2017.
Balch CM, Buzaid AC, Soong SJ, et al. Final version of the American Joint Committee on Cancer staging system for cutaneous melanoma. J Clin Oncol 2001;19(16):3635–48.
Balch CM, Gerschenwald JE, Soong SJ, et al. Multivariate analysis of prognostic factors among 2313 patients with stage III melanoma: comparison of nodal micrometastases versus macrometastases. J Clin Oncol 2010;28(14):2452–9.
Balch CM, Gershenwald JE, Soong SJ, et al. Final version of 2009 AJCC melanoma staging and classification. J Clin Oncol 2009;27(36):6199–206.
Balch CM, Morton DL, Gershenwald JE, et al. Sentinel node biopsy and standard of care for melanoma. J Am Acad Dermatol 2009;60(5):872–5.

Balch CM, Soong SJ, Gershenwald JE, et al. Prognostic factors analysis of 17,600 melanoma patients: validation of the American Joint Committee on Cancer melanoma staging system. J Clin Oncol 2001;19(16):3622–34.

Bichakjian CK, Hapern AC, Johnson TM, et al. Guidelines of care for the management of primary cutaneous melanoma. American Academy of Dermatology. J Am Acad Dermatol 2011;65(5):1032–47.

Buzaid AC, Rossi MI, Balch CM, et al. Critical analysis of the current American Joint Committee on Cancer staging system for cutaneous melanoma and proposal of a new staging system. J Clin Oncol 1997;15(3):1039–51.

Lee CC, Faries MB, Wanek LA, Morton DL. Improved survival after lymphadenectomy for nodal metastasis from an unknown primary melanoma. J Clin Oncol 2008;26(4):535–41.

Carlson GW, Murray DR, Hestley A, Staley CA, Lyles RH, Cohen C. Sentinel lymph node mapping for thick (> or =4 mm) melanoma: should we be doing it? Ann Surg Oncol 2003;10(4):408–15.

Cascinelli N, Belli F, Santinami M, et al. Sentinel lymph node biopsy in cutaneous melanoma: the WHO Melanoma Program experience. Ann Surg Oncol 2000;7(6):469–74.

Cascinelli N, Bombardieri E, Bufalino R, et al. Sentinel and nonsentinel node status in stage IB and II melanoma patients: two-step prognostic indicators of survival. J Clin Oncol 2006;24(27):4464–71.

Cavanaugh-Hussey MW, Mu EW, Kang S, Balch CM, Wang T. Older age is associated with a higher incidence of sentinel lymph node metastasis death but a lower incidence of sentinel lymph node metastasis in the SEER databases (2003–2011). Ann Surg Oncol 2015;22(7):2120–6.

Clark PB, Soo V, Kraas J, Shen P, Levine EA. Futility of fluorodeoxyglucose F-18 positron emission tomography in initial evaluation of patients with T2 to T4 melanoma. Arch Surg 2006;141(3):284–8.

Cormier JN, Xing Y, Feng L, et al. Metastatic melanoma to lymph nodes in patients with unknown primary sites. Cancer 2006;106(9):2012–20.

Gajdos C, Griffith KA, Wong SL, et al. Is there a benefit to sentinel lymph node biopsy in patients with T4 melanoma? Cancer 2009;115(24):5752–60.

Gimotty PA, Elder DE, Fraket DL, et al. Identification of high-risk patients among those diagnosed with thin cutaneous melanomas. J Clin Oncol 2007;25(9):1129–34.

Macdonald JB, Dueck AC, Gray RJ, et al. Malignant melanoma in the elderly: different regional disease and poorer prognosis. J Cancer 2011;2:538–43.

Maubec E, Lumbroso J, Masson F, et al. F-18 fluorodeoxy-D-glucose positron emission tomography scan in the initial evaluation of patients with a primary melanoma thicker than 4 mm. Melanoma Res 2007;17(3):147–54.

Mills JK, White I, Diggs B, Fortino J, Vetto JT. Effect of biopsy type on outcomes in the treatment of primary cutaneous melanoma. Am J Surg 2013;205(5):585–90.

Miranda EP, Gertner M, Wall J, et al. Routine imaging of asymptomatic melanoma patients with metastasis to sentinel lymph node rarely identifies systemic disease. Arch Surg 2004;139(8):831–6.

Mu E, Lange JR, Strouse JJ. Comparison of the use and results of sentinel lymph node biopsy in children and young adults with melanoma. Cancer 2012;118(10):2700–7.

National Collaborating Centre for Cancer (NCC-C). Melanoma: assessment and management. London, UK: National Institute for Health and care Excellence; 2015.

National Comprehensive Cancer Network. <http://www.nccn.org/professionals/physicians_gls/f_guidelines.asp>; 2011.

Page AJ, Li A, Hestley A, Murray D, Carlson GW, Delman KA. Increasing age is associated with worse prognostic factors and increased distant recurrences despite fewer sentinel lymph node positives in melanoma. Int J Surg Oncol 2012;2012:456987.

Slade AD, Austin MT. Childhood melanoma: an increasingly important health problem in the USA. Curr Opin Pediatr 2014;26(3):356–61.

Ulrich J, van Akkooi AJ, Eggermont AM, Voit C. New developments in melanoma: utility of ultrasound imaging (initial staging, follow-up and pre-SLNB). Expert Rev Anticancer Ther 2011;11(11):1693–701.

Wagner JD, Schauwecker D, Davidson D, et al. Inefficacy of F-18 fluorodeoxy-D-glucose-positron emission tomography scans for initial evaluation in early-stage cutaneous melanoma. Cancer 2005;104(3):570–9.

Wasif N, Etzioni D, Haddad D, Gray RJ, Bagaria SP, Pockaj BA. Staging studies for cutaneous melanoma in the United States: a population-based analysis. Ann Surg Oncol 2015;22(4):1366–70.

Weiss SA, Hanniford D, Hernando E, Osman I. Revisiting determinants of prognosis in cutaneous melanoma. Cancer 2015;121:4108–23.

Yancovitz M, Finelt N, Warycha MA, et al. Role of radiologic imaging at the time of initial diagnosis of stage T1b–T3b melanoma. Cancer 2007;110(5):1107–14.

Therapy of Melanoma

Cutaneous Melanoma. http://dx.doi.org/10.1016/B978-0-12-804000-3.00005-3

SUBCHAPTER

5.1

Stage 0–2

Susana Puig*,**, Sergi Vidal-Sicart*,**, Antoni Bennassar*,**, Josep Malvehy*,**

*University of Barcelona, Barcelona, Spain
**Research Center of the Biomedical Network of Rare Diseases (CIBERER), Carlos III Health Institute, Madrid, Spain

1 INTRODUCTION

The treatment of the primary tumor aims to eliminate the lesions with safety margins, to decrease the risk of relapse, and to better characterize the prognosis of the disease.

2 SURGICAL THERAPY

2.1 Margins

The surgical treatment of the primary tumor aims to excise the complete lesion with safety margins that minimize the risk of local recurrence.

Radial margins recommended (T AJCC staging 2009 and guideline recommendations [1–3]) are as follows:

- 0.5 cm in melanoma in situ
- 1 cm in invasive melanoma <2 mm thickness
- 2 cm in invasive melanoma >2 mm thickness
  - Recurrence rate for thin melanomas (<1 mm) is less than 2%, being associated with lentigo maligna melanoma (Figs. 5.1.1–5.1.10), acral melanoma, desmoplastic melanoma, and <8-mm histological margins (corresponding to <10-mm surgical margins) [2].

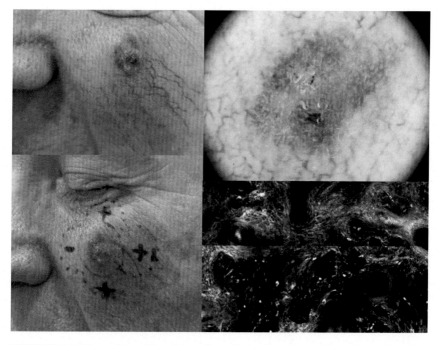

FIGURE 5.1.1 **Lentigo maligna melanoma on the left cheek that under dermoscopy shows an unspecific global pattern, with multiple colors and shiny white streaks.** Reflectance confocal microscopy shows atypical basal cells and atypical cells in the upper dermis in normal-appearing skin allowing a better margin delimitation before surgery.

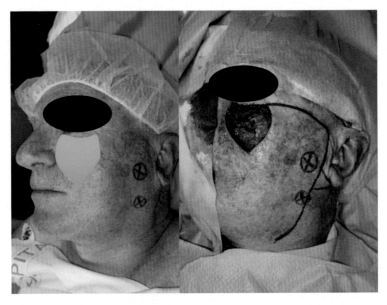

FIGURE 5.1.2   **Same patient.** Wide excision of the melanoma and surgical reconstruction.

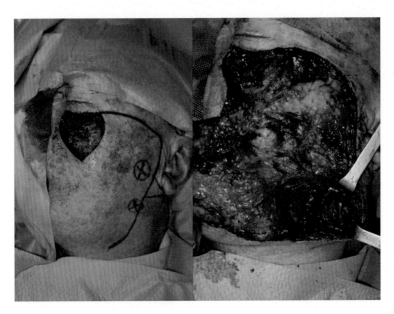

FIGURE 5.1.3   **Same patient.** Identification of the two sentinel lymph nodes.

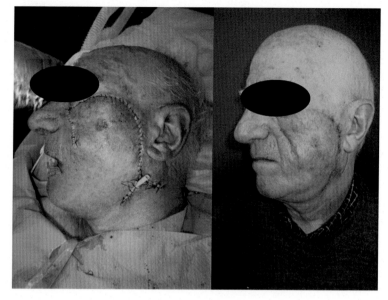

FIGURE 5.1.4 **Same patient.** Postsurgical closure and result after 3 months.

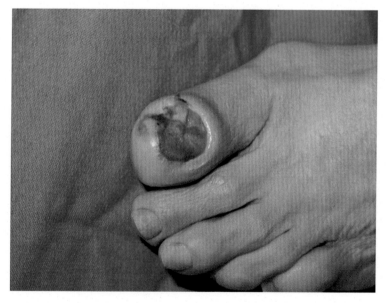

FIGURE 5.1.5 **Amelanotic nail matrix invasive melanoma (>1 mm thickness).**

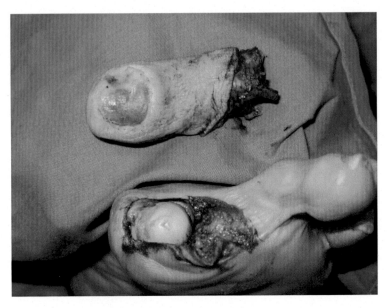

FIGURE 5.1.6 **Same patient.** Disarticulation of the toe.

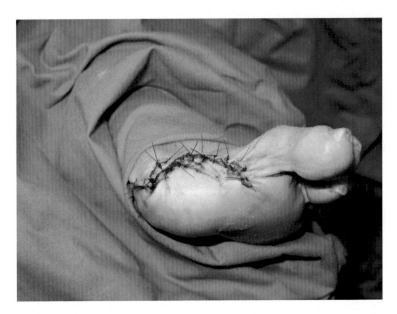

FIGURE 5.1.7 **Same patient.** Surgical closure.

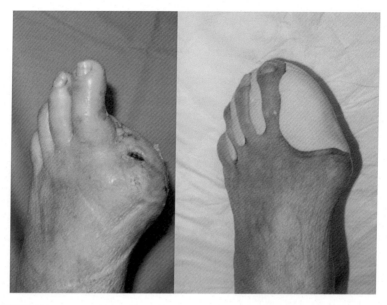

FIGURE 5.1.8 **Same patient.** Result after 3 months and prosthesis to improve physiology of standing up and walking.

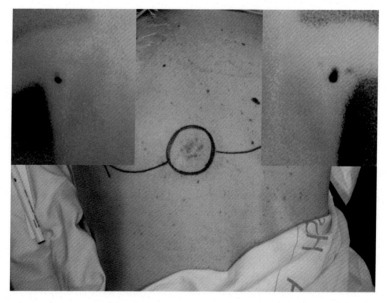

FIGURE 5.1.9 **Planning of wide excision of melanoma on the back with bilateral lymphatic drainage in the lymphography.**

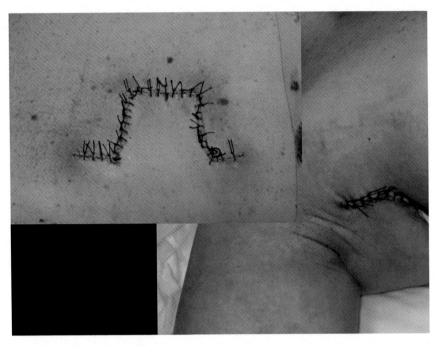

FIGURE 5.1.10 **Same patient.** Surgical closure of the wide excision on the back and incision for sentinel lymph node biopsy in the axilla.

- Long-term retrospective studies did not demonstrate any differences in recurrence rate, local metastases, or overall survival (OS) between 1- and 2-cm margins in melanomas thicker than 2 mm [4].
- However, a recent metaanalysis suggests that wide margins (2 cm) could be associated with lower melanoma-specific mortality [5].

2.2 Special Locations

Wide margin excision is not always feasible.

- Large lentigo malignant melanomas of face: They may be excised with narrow margins [6] without increasing the local recurrence rate.
  - If narrow or positive margins: adjuvant radiotherapy (RT) or topical agents (imiquimod) [7,8]
- Mucosal melanoma: Margins may be reduced to anatomical limits [6].
- Nail melanoma: The complete matricectomy is necessary.
  - In in situ and early invasive melanoma (<0.75 mm), amputation of the distal phalange is not recommended [9,10].
- Acral melanoma: Amputation is not recommended but occasionally needed in fingers if thick, large, and ulcerated melanomas are present [1].

3 ADJUVANT THERAPY

A very low number of melanoma patients can benefit from adjuvant therapy nowadays. For more than 20 years interferon has been the only approved adjuvant treatment that demonstrated a moderate increased disease-free survival (DFS) but small benefit in OS compared with placebo [11–18].

3.1 Interferon

- Two different protocols: low or high doses (Table 5.1.1):
  - Equally effective in terms of DFS
  - Benefit in terms of OS only in trials with low-dose interferon, namely, 3 MU subcutaneous 3 days a week for 36 months:
    - This finding is in contrast with the common belief in the United States that high-dose interferon is the most effective.
- Best efficacy reached in ulcerated, stage 2 primary melanoma [16]

3.2 Vaccines

- Not superior to placebo or other therapies [13,19–22]

3.3 Immunotherapy

- Ipilimumab (anti–CTLA-4 antibody) demonstrated superiority in DFS compared with placebo in high-risk stage III melanoma patients, 3-year recurrence-free survival being 46.5% (95% CI 41.5–51.3) in the

TABLE 5.1.1 More Commonly Used Schedules for Adjuvant Treatment With Interferon Alpha-2b in High-Risk Melanoma Patients

High dose	Induction: interferon alpha-2b 20 MU/m^2 intravenously over 20 min daily for 5 consecutive days for 4 weeks Maintenance: interferon alpha-2b 10 MU/m^2 subcutaneous 3 days a week for 11 months
Medium dose	Interferon alpha-2b 5–10 MU/m^2 subcutaneous 3 days a week for 18 months
Low dose	Interferon alpha-2b 1–3 MU subcutaneous 3 days a week for 18–36 months
Peg-intron	Pegylated interferon alfa-2b 100 µg subcutaneous once weekly for 36 months

ipilimumab group versus 34.8% (95% CI 30.1–39.5) in the placebo group [23] and the median recurrence-free survival was 26.1 months (95% CI 19.3–39.3) in the ipilimumab group versus 17.1 months (95% CI 13.4–21.6) in the placebo group (hazard ratio 0.75; 95% CI 0.64–0.90; $P = 0.0013$) [23].

- Unfortunately, this benefit was associated with serious toxicity and some deaths.
- Best efficacy is reached in stage 3C melanoma with four or more positive lymph nodes.

- Several trials are investigating the benefits of BRAF inhibitors alone or associated with MEK inhibitors in adjuvant treatment of *BRAF* mutant melanoma patients free of disease after surgery (https://clinicaltrials.gov). Finally, several trials are investigating the use of anti–PD-1 drugs in adjuvancy (pembrolizumab and nivolumab) (https://clinicaltrials.gov).

4 MEDICAL THERAPY

In some cases, when complete excision could be difficult or associated with high morbidity or high risk to leave affected margins, other therapeutic options can be considered.

4.1 Topical Imiquimod

- In LM 70% of complete responses are confirmed by reflectance confocal microscopy and biopsies [24,25].
- Combination of tazarotene and imiquimod seems to increase the number of complete responses [26].

4.2 Radiotherapy

- In LM the cure rates achieved (with either Grenz rays or soft X-rays using the Miescher technique) range from 86 to 95%:
  - Potential second-line treatment
  - Usually reserved for nonsurgical lesions in elderly
  - Grenz ray therapy (12 kV) (100–120 Gy; 10 Gy twice weekly for 5–6 weeks [27])
- It is proposed in desmoplastic melanoma when narrowed margins, high-risk locations, or other risk factors are present:
  - In desmoplastic melanomas when surgery is not possible, electrochemotherapy has been reported as an alternative local treatment [28] with control of the local diseases.

5 CONCLUSIONS

The treatment of primary melanoma is mainly surgical with wide margins of the primary tumor (adequate to the T AJCC staging). The only approved adjuvant treatment for melanoma is interferon alpha with limited benefits and manageable toxicities. Nevertheless, target immunotherapy with ipilimumab already showed benefits in adjuvant setting but was associated with serious toxicity. Other treatments such as RT or local treatments can be considered in special locations and situations but should be better discussed in a melanoma conference with a multidisciplinary team and adapt to the conditions of the patient.

References

[1] Garbe C, Peris K, Hauschild A, Saiag P, Middleton M, Spatz A, et al. Diagnosis and treatment of melanoma. European consensus-based interdisciplinary guideline—update 2012. Eur J Cancer 2012;48(15):2375–90.

[2] MacKenzie Ross AD, Haydu LE, Quinn MJ, Saw RPM, Shannon KF, Spillane AJ, et al. The association between excision margins and local recurrence in 11,290 thin (T1) primary cutaneous melanomas: a case–control study. Ann Surg Oncol 2016;23:1082–9.

[3] National Comprehensive Cancer Network. NCCN clinical practice guidelines in oncology, <http://www.nccn.org/professionals/physician_gls/f_guidelines.asp#site>; 2014.

[4] Hunger RE, Angermeier S, Seyed Jafari SM, Ochsenbein A, Shafighi M. A retrospective study of 1- versus 2-cm excision margins for cutaneous malignant melanomas thicker than 2 mm. J Am Acad Dermatol 2015;72(6):1054–9.

[5] Wheatley K, Wilson JS, Gaunt P, Marsden JR. Surgical excision margins in primary cutaneous melanoma: a meta-analysis and Bayesian probability evaluation. Cancer Treat Rev 2016;42:73–81.

[6] Rawlani R, Rawlani V, Qureshi HA, Kim JY, Wayne JD. Reducing margins of wide local excision in head and neck melanoma for function and cosmesis: 5-year local recurrence-free survival. J Surg Oncol 2015;111(7):795–9.

[7] Read T, Noonan C, David M, Wagels M, Foote M, Schaider H, et al. A systematic review of non-surgical treatments for lentigo maligna. J Eur Acad Dermatol Venereol 2016;30:748–53.

[8] Pandit AS, Geiger EJ, Ariyan S, Narayan D, Choi JN. Using topical imiquimod for the management of positive in situ margins after melanoma resection. Cancer Med 2015;4(4):507–12.

[9] Duarte AF, Correia O, Barros AM, Ventura F, Haneke E. Nail melanoma in situ: clinical, dermoscopic, pathologic clues, and steps for minimally invasive treatment. Dermatol Surg 2015;41(1):59–68.

[10] Debarbieux S, Gaspar R, Depaepe L, Dalle S, Balme B, Thomas L. Intraoperative diagnosis of nonpigmented nail tumours with ex vivo fluorescence confocal microscopy: 10 cases. Br J Dermatol 2015;172(4):1037–44.

[11] Kirkwood JM, Strawderman MH, Ernstoff MS, Smith TJ, Borden EC, Blum RH. Interferon alfa-2b adjuvant therapy of high-risk resected cutaneous melanoma: the Eastern Cooperative Oncology Group Trial EST 1684. J Clin Oncol 1996;14(1):7–17.

[12] Kirkwood JM, Ibrahim JG, Sondak VK, Richards J, Flaherty LE, Ernstoff MS, et al. High- and low-dose interferon alfa-2b in high-risk melanoma: first analysis of intergroup trial E1690/S9111/C9190. J Clin Oncol 2000;18(12):2444–58.

[13] Kirkwood BJM, Ibrahim JG, Sosman JA, Sondak VK, Agarwala SS, Ernstoff MS. High-dose interferon alfa-2b significantly prolongs relapse-free and overall survival compared with the GM2-KLH/QS-21 vaccine in patients with resected stage IIB–III melanoma: results of intergroup trial. J Clin Oncol 2001;19(9):2370–80.

[14] Kirkwood JM, Manola J, Ibrahim J, Sondak V, Ernstoff MS, Rao U. A pooled analysis of Eastern Cooperative Oncology Group and intergroup trials of adjuvant high-dose interferon for melanoma. Clin Cancer Res 2004;10(412):1670–7.

[15] Pehamberger H, Soyer HP, Steiner A, Kofler R, Binder M, Mischer P, et al. Adjuvant interferon alfa-2a treatment in resected primary stage II cutaneous melanoma. Austrian Malignant Melanoma Cooperative Group. J Clin Oncol 1998;16:1425–9.

[16] Eggermont AMM, Suciu S, Testori A, Kruit WH, Marsden J, Punt CJ, et al. Ulceration and stage are predictive of interferon efficacy in melanoma: results of the phase III adjuvant trials EORTC 18952 and EORTC 18991. Eur J Cancer 2012;48(2):218–25.

[17] Eggermont AMM, Suciu S, Rutkowski P, Kruit WH, Punt CJ, Dummer R, et al. Long term follow up of the EORTC 18952 trial of adjuvant therapy in resected stage IIB–III cutaneous melanoma patients comparing intermediate doses of interferon-alpha-2b (IFN) with observation: ulceration of primary is key determinant for IFN-sensitivity. Eur J Cancer 2016;55:111–21.

[18] Grob JJ, Jouary T, Dréno B, Asselineau J, Gutzmer R, Hauschild A, et al. Adjuvant therapy with pegylated interferon alfa-2b (36 months) versus low-dose interferon alfa-2b (18 months) in melanoma patients without macrometastatic nodes: an open-label, randomised, phase 3 European Association for Dermato-Oncology (EADO) study. Eur J Cancer 2013;49(1):166–74.

[19] Vilella R, Benítez D, Milà J, Lozano M, Vilana R, Pomes J, et al. Pilot study of treatment of biochemotherapy-refractory stage IV melanoma patients with autologous dendritic cells pulsed with a heterologous melanoma cell line lysate. Cancer Immunol Immunother 2004;53(7):651–8.

[20] Vilella R, Benitez D, Milà J, Vilalta A, Rull R, Cuellar F, et al. Treatment of patients with progressive unresectable metastatic melanoma with a heterologous polyvalent melanoma whole cell vaccine. Int J Cancer 2003;106(4):626–31.

[21] Ridolfi L, Petrini M, Fiammenghi L, Granato AM, Ancarani V, Pancisi E, et al. Dendritic cell-based vaccine in advanced melanoma: update of clinical outcome. Melanoma Res 2011;21(6):524–9.

[22] Hodi S. Improved survival with ipilimumab in patients with metastatic melanoma. N Engl J Med 2010;609–19.

[23] Eggermont AMM, Chiarion-Sileni V, Grob J-J, Dummer R, Wolchok JD, Schmidt H, et al. Adjuvant ipilimumab versus placebo after complete resection of high-risk stage III melanoma (EORTC 18071): a randomised, double-blind, phase 3 trial. Lancet Oncol 2015;16(5):522–30.

[24] Tzellos T, Kyrgidis A, Mocellin S, Chan A-W, Pilati P, Apalla Z. Interventions for melanoma in situ, including lentigo maligna. Cochrane Database Syst Rev 2014;12(12). CD010308.

[25] Alarcon I, Carrera C, Alos L, Palou J, Malvehy J, Puig S. In vivo reflectance confocal microscopy to monitor the response of lentigo maligna to imiquimod. J Am Acad Dermatol 2014;71(1):49–55.

[26] Hyde MA, Hadley ML, Tristani-Firouzi P, Goldgar D, Bowen GM. A randomized trial of the off-label use of imiquimod, 5%, cream with vs without tazarotene, 0.1%, gel for the treatment of lentigo maligna, followed by conservative staged excisions. Arch Dermatol 2012;148(5):592–6.

[27] Garbe C, Schadendorf D, Stolz W, Volkenandt M, Reinhold U, Kortmann R-D, et al. Short German guidelines: malignant melanoma. J Dtsch Dermatol Ges 2008;6(Suppl. 1): S9–S14.

[28] Carrera C, Bennassar A, Ishioka P, Dalle S, Vilalta A, Fuertes I, et al. Desmoplastic melanoma on the nose: electrochemotherapy as an alternative treatment to local advanced disease. J Eur Acad Dermatol Venereol 2014;28:424–32.

Further Reading

Morton DL, Thompson JF, Cochran AJ, Mozzillo N, Elashoff R, Essner R, et al. Sentinel-node biopsy or nodal observation in melanoma. N Engl J Med 2006;355(13):1307–17.

Morton DL, Thompson JF, Cochran AJ, Mozzillo N, Nieweg OE, Roses DF, et al. Final trial report of sentinel-node biopsy versus nodal observation in melanoma. N Engl J Med 2014;370(7):599–609.

Balch CM, Gershenwald JE, Soong S-J, Thompson JF, Atkins MB, Byrd DR, et al. Final version of 2009 AJCC melanoma staging and classification. J Clin Oncol 2009;27(36):6199–206.

Mocellin S, Lens MB, Pasquali S, Pilati P, Chiarion Sileni V. Interferon alpha for the adjuvant treatment of cutaneous melanoma. Cochrane Database Syst Rev 2013;(6). CD008955.

Malczewski A, Marshall A, Payne MJ, Mao L, Bafaloukos D, Si L, et al. Intravenous high-dose interferon with or without maintenance treatment in melanoma at high risk of recurrence: meta-analysis of three trials. Cancer Med 2016;5(1):17–23.

Guitera P, Haydu LE, Menzies SW, Scolyer RA, Hong A, Fogarty GB, et al. Surveillance for treatment failure of lentigo maligna with dermoscopy and *in vivo* confocal microscopy: new descriptors. Br J Dermatol 2014;170(6):1305–12.

SUBCHAPTER

5.2

Treatment of Stage III Melanoma

Mario Santinami, Gianfrancesco Gallino, Ilaria Mattavelli,
Roberto Patuzzo, Andrea Maurichi

IRCCS Foundation of the National Cancer Institute, Milan, Italy

Cutaneous melanoma at stage III expresses a locoregional spread of disease that may be characterized by lymph node metastases and/or in-transit metastases (IT-mets).

1 TREATMENT OF LYMPH NODE METASTASES

1.1 Lymph Node Metastases

- Metastases to regional lymph nodes represent the most important prognostic factor in melanoma patients and generally occur in 20% of cases [1,2].

- Sentinel node biopsy (SNB) allows to early identify patients with occult disease who may benefit from an immediate lymph node dissection, in order to improve disease-free survival (DFS) and melanoma-specific survival (MSS) [3–11].
  - The gold standard of treatment for a node-positive disease is the complete dissection of the lymph node basin involved. It is defined as follows:
    - Completion lymph node dissection (CLND): When it is performed after a positive SNB, in order to complete the removal of the remaining non–sentinel nodes (SNs)
    - Therapeutic lymph node dissection (TLND): When it is performed after a clinical or radiological detection of metastatic nodes, confirmed after a histological examination
- However, numerous controversial issues on this topic do exist:
  - The management of melanoma nodal metastases, detected after a positive SNB, with a CLND is still debated (benefits vs. the side effects).
    - Findings supporting a routine CLND are as follows:
      - Some investigations did not identify relevant subpopulations of patients having a low risk of further metastatic non-SNs [12,13].
      - Histological analysis of non-SNs is typically less accurate as compared to that of SNs, so that the detection of metastatic cells in non-SNs could be underestimated; this may impact on patient outcome, since the detection of metastatic non-SNs is associated with an unfavorable prognosis [14].
      - The Multicenter Selective Lymphadenectomy Trial (MSLT-I) indicated that SN-positive patients in the SNB arm who underwent early CLND had less morbidity than patients in the observation arm who underwent delayed TLND at the time of nodal recurrence [15]. Moreover, SN-positive patients who underwent early CLND had higher survival rates than those with delayed TLND at the time of metastatic nodal recurrence, particularly for primary melanoma of intermediate thickness [11,16].
      - The most important side effects deriving from a CLND (including edema, lymphorrhea, etc.) are associated with the superficial inguinal–crural dissection rather than the deep iliac–obturatory dissection. In addition, this procedure shows a higher morbidity when delayed until a clinical or radiological evidence of disease nodal relapse occurs. The increased morbidity recorded for a delayed CLND suggests to adopt this procedure in cases of positive SNB rather than in those of macroscopic nodal disease.

- Findings not supporting a routine CLND are as follows:
  - Not all patients with positive SNs develop clinical regional recurrence; in some cases the metastatic deposit in the SN represents the initial expression of the spread of disease, while in others the SNB may have removed the only metastatic focus. Thus, routine CLND in all SN-positive cases could lead to overtreatment for a subgroup of patients, while another subset will achieve a real benefit.
  - Results showing that CLND could improve survival as compared to a clinic and radiological observation after the detection of positive SNs are lacking; the hypothesis that the clinical nodal observation associated with a regular ultrasonography could be an acceptable procedure for patients with positive SNs is currently under prospective investigation in the randomized MSLT-II [17], but answering this question will require many years of follow-up.
  - A recent study found no benefit of complete lymph node dissection compared with that of observation in patients with melanoma and micrometastases in the sentinel lymph node. Therefore, complete lymphadenectomy should not be recommended in patients with melanoma with micrometastasis, at least in those with single cells or micrometastases of 1 mm diameter or less.
- The optimal extent of the groin lymph node dissection for melanoma patients with positive SNB is another debated issue.
  - No agreement exists with regard to the surgical removal of pelvic (iliac–obturatory) lymph nodes.
    - Given the reported morbidity, including wound infection, seroma, flap necrosis, and lymph edema up to 80%, some surgeons consider the benefit–risk ratio unfavorable for patients, and thus limit the completion lymphadenectomy to the inguinal–crural nodal basin.
    - Conversely, other surgeons consider the incidence of pelvic lymph node metastases a relevant risk, sufficient to perform the pelvic completion lymphadenectomy, too. Such an aggressive approach may also be driven by the low benefits deriving from the approved codified adjuvant treatments, particularly from the use of interferon (IFN)-alpha [18].
    - In addition, a multicentric study showed that pelvic lymph nodes are frequently positive after an iliac–obturatory dissection.
  - Since the pelvic lymph node metastases were associated with a worse prognosis, pelvic lymph nodes should always be considered [19].

- Another key question open to discussion concerns the prognostic value of metastatic deposit in SN.
  - The SN tumor burden is considered a significant prognostic factor for patient survival [20] [5-year overall survival (OS) rate of 100% in patients with single cell metastatic involvement of the SN, and 5-year distant metastasis-free survival of 91%, in line with the rates found in the SN-negative patient group].
    - Submicrometastasis (<0.1 mm) involvement of SN or isolated cluster of melanoma cells (>10) could biologically be considered differently from larger micrometastatic disease, and patients who showed this micrometastatic involvement in their regional nodes could be spared the morbidity of a CLND without compromising their survival chances.
    - Subsequent analyses [21–23] investigated different prognostic factors, particularly among cases with nodal metastatic deposit <0.1 mm, and showed that, when it was located in the subcapsular area, patients may be overtreated by a CLND, since their survival rates were similar to those of SN-negative patients.
- Up to date, the joint ASCO–SSO guidelines recommend as standard of care a CLND for all patients with positive SN [24,25].

1.2 Surgical Approach to Regional Lymph Node Basins

The cervical, axillar, and inguinal–iliac regional nodal basins are those generally involved by metastatic disease and candidate to surgery. Less frequently, the epitrochlear and popliteal basins are interested by metastatic spread.

1.2.1 Cervical Lymph Node Dissection (Fig. 5.2.1)

- The cervical node basin receives metastatic cells from primary head, neck, and upper trunk cancers.
- The surgical approach to patients with positive lymph nodes in this region is generally a modified neck dissection that includes the II, III, IV, and V levels, preserving the spinal accessory nerve, the internal jugular vein, and the sternocleidomastoid muscle.
- A concomitant superficial parotidectomy is usually performed in case of primary melanomas on the frontal scalp or temporal regions with a lymphatic spread to the parotid.
- The importance of the number of removed nodes in this kind of dissection has to be underlined; a cervical lymph node dissection including 4 or more levels should remove at least 20 lymph nodes [19].
- A radical neck dissection must be performed in case of evidence of macroscopic nodal disease in this anatomic area.

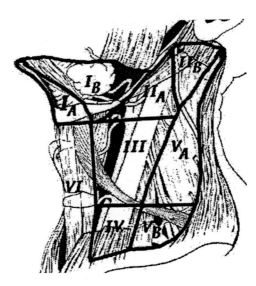

FIGURE 5.2.1 **Neck dissection.**

1.2.2 *Axillary Lymph Node Dissection (Fig. 5.2.2)*

- A complete axillary lymphadenectomy must include the removal of I, II, and III nodal levels in association with the minor pectoralis muscle.
- Also for this area the optimal number of excised lymph nodes is at least 20 [19].
- The evidence that only 18%–20% of these patients have further metastatic nodes at the CLND opened a discussion on the dissection of the axillary level III nodes.

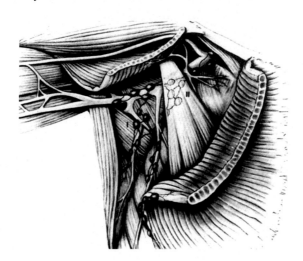

FIGURE 5.2.2 **Axillary dissection.**

- However, to date the standard recommendations remain a complete dissection including the axillary III nodal levels.

1.2.3 Inguinal–Crural (Superficial) and Iliac–Obturatory (Deep) Lymph Node Dissection (Fig. 5.2.3)

- Patients with inguinal nodal metastatic disease should undergo either superficial (inguinal–crural) dissection or deep (iliac–obturatory) dissection.
- This procedure must include the removal of the Cloquet node that is localized within the pelvis posteriorly and medially to the external iliac vein. The femoral nerve, running along the medial portion of the sartorius muscle, should be preserved while the saphenous vein is ligated at the level of the saphenofemoral junction and the femoral artery and vein are skeletonized.
- Iliac-obturatory lymph node dissection via a lateral abdominal extraperitoneal approach. The ureter is identified and preserved, while the epigastric vessels are ligated and the external iliac vessels are visualized and skeletonized up to the bifurcation of the common iliac vessels. The obturator nerve is identified and preserved and

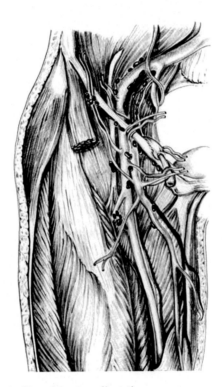

FIGURE 5.2.3   Groin iliac–obturatory dissection.

finally the sartorius muscle is disengaged and rotated to cover and protect the femoral vessel.

- In this kind of dissection, the optimal number of removed lymph nodes could range between 15 and 25 [19].
- However, some surgeons perform only a superficial dissection in patients for whom there is an evidence of an inguinal microscopic nodal disease (SN-positive), although this procedure is not recommended due to the frequent detection of further positive pelvic nodes after the iliac–obturatory dissection [19].

1.2.4 Lymph Node Dissection of Minor Basins

- The presence of metastatic nodal disease can be detected after a SNB or a clinical/radiological exam also in minor nodal basins, such as the popliteal and epitrochlear ones.
- In similar cases, the therapeutic indication consists in the removal of all the lymph nodes lying in those areas.

2 ADJUVANT THERAPY

Metastases to the regional lymph nodes are the most common first clinical manifestation of disease spread after the excision of the primary tumor or for unknown primary melanoma [26]. Systemic adjuvant therapy has been investigated over the past decades in stage III melanoma patients with high risk of relapse, due to the poor effectiveness of surgical treatment alone.

2.1 Interferon

- To date, IFN is the only approved agent for an adjuvant therapy of stage III melanoma in patients who had already undergone surgery and with high risk of recurrence.
- In particular, IFN alfa-2b was approved in Europe and the United States, the pegylated (Peg) form of IFN alfa-2b in the United States and Switzerland, and the IFN alfa-2a in Europe. The mechanism of action of IFN in melanoma appears to be mainly immunomodulatory, although it also has an antiproliferative activity [27–29].
- Many dose regimens have been tested over the years and metaanalyses of phase III trials demonstrated that IFN has a consistent effect on recurrence-free survival (RFS) and DFS, but none or very low effect on OS [30–35]. These findings suggest that only a few subsets of patients are sensitive to IFN.
- These trials stratified patients by SN staging and by the presence or absence of ulceration in the primary tumor.

- Both stage and ulceration emerged as prognostic factors; in fact, patients with nodal micrometastases and nonulcerated primary tumors had a better prognosis than those with clinically detected node metastases and ulceration in the primary lesion [1,2].
- There is no definitive evidence regarding the optimal dose and duration of therapy with this agent. The overall clinical evidence should be shared with melanoma patients with an intermediate–high risk of relapse after surgery and a discussion on the advantages and disadvantages of different regimens, including potential side effects, should support the decision of using IFN as an adjuvant agent.

2.2 The MAGE Protein Family

- Several immunotherapy strategies have recently shown that immune manipulation can mediate regression of malignancies. The discovery of tumor antigens and of T lymphocytes directed against them has provided the basis for antigen-specific immunotherapy [36].
- In the past decade, several vaccination strategies have been designed for different treatments.
- The MAGE-A3 gene is expressed during embryogenesis and in a great variety of tumors [37]. It is presented to specific T cells by HLA molecules at the cell surface as a tumor-specific antigen [38], while it is not expressed in normal adult tissues, except testis and placenta [39]. Thus, this represented a selective target for tumor-specific active immunotherapy.
- Pilot studies [40,41] showed that immunotherapy with recombinant MAGE-A3 protein had antitumor activity in patients with metastatic melanoma, with a good tolerability.
  - However, the preliminary evidence from a recent randomized trial showed that this therapeutic approach did not improve patient survival.

2.3 BRAF and NRAS Inhibitors

- The constitutive hyperactivation of the RAS/RAF/MEK/ERK pathway has been identified as the regulator of cell proliferation, invasion, and survival of melanocytic cells [42–46].
- The frequency of BRAF mutations varies between 40 and 70% in cutaneous melanoma [43,44,47], while NRAS mutations are present in 15%–30% of cutaneous melanomas [48,49].
- Many clinical trials are still testing the effectiveness and safety of these molecules in melanoma patients with intermediate/advanced disease. The first agent to be studied was vemurafenib. After the results of

clinical trials, this molecule was approved for treatment of metastatic melanoma [50]. Another BRAF inhibitor used for adjuvant treatment of stage III melanoma at high risk of recurrence is dabrafenib, approved as a single agent in the treatment of metastatic disease with BRAF V600E mutation [51–55]. The combination dabrafenib–trametinib was used as adjuvant therapy in stage III melanoma patients with BRAF V600E or K mutation. The combination of these targeted agents produced additive effects, but resistances occurred in most patients, with a short period of tumor control [56].

2.4 Anti–CTLA-4

- Longer responses in time seem to depend on immunologic control and are rarely obtained with chemotherapy or targeted therapies alone. This was first demonstrated by the effectiveness of anti–CTLA-4 molecules, resulting in the approval of ipilimumab, a monoclonal antibody against CTLA-4, for patients with advanced melanoma [57,58].
- The results of a recent randomized controlled trial evaluating the impact of adjuvant ipilimumab versus placebo in patients with advanced stage III melanoma indicated a significant impact on RFS (median RFS was 17 months in the placebo arm vs. 26 months in the treatment arm).
- As compared to targeted agents in BRAF-mutated melanomas, response rates with ipilimumab were slightly lower (i.e., $-10/-15\%$), but had longer durability (i.e., about 1.5–2 years) in melanoma mutated and nonmutated patients [57,58]. Recent results confirmed that immunotherapy with ipilimumab is associated with 2- to 5-year survival in about 20% of previously treated patients and in over 30% of naive ones [59].
- Adverse events were quite frequent, often with grade 3–4, and were generally immune-related. Most adverse events involved the gastrointestinal, hepatic, and endocrine systems, and most of them were managed and resolved.

2.5 Anti–PD-1/PD-L1

- The programmed death (PD)-1 receptor represents another key immune receptor expressed by activated T cells [60,61].
- The efficacy of the anti–PD-1 molecules nivolumab and pembrolizumab appears better than that of ipilimumab; response rates were higher, ranging from 30% to 50%. The durability of response is similar or longer than that induced by ipilimumab, and the toxicity profile is also much more favorable [62–64].

- High expression of PD-L1 on tumor cells is associated with a worse prognosis and survival in several kinds of cancers such as renal cell, pancreatic, hepatocellular, and ovarian carcinomas [65–68]. Recent data from a phase III trial showed better results in terms of effectiveness of pembrolizumab versus that of ipilimumab. The estimated 6-month progression-free survival (PFS) rates were 47.3% for pembrolizumab administered every 2 weeks, 46.4% for pembrolizumab administered every 3 weeks, and 26.5% for ipilimumab. The corresponding 12-month survival rates were 74.1, 68.4, and 58.2% [69].

In conclusion, the prognosis for patients with melanoma has improved radically over the past few years. The therapeutic approaches in use, as well as the availability of new molecules for adjuvant treatments in patients with stage III melanoma with high risk of recurrence after surgery, are becoming even more promising.

3 TREATMENT OF IN-TRANSIT METASTASES

3.1 In-Transit Metastases

- Five to 8% of melanoma patients will develop IT-mets.
- These lesions are tumor embolic expressions within the dermal and subdermal lymphatics and can occur between the site of the primary tumor and the draining regional lymph nodal basin.
- IT-mets often anticipate the appearance of systemic disease and are associated with 5-year survival rates of 69 and 52%, respectively, depending on the concomitant absence or presence of lymph node metastases [1].
- Various treatment options exist according to the presentation and can range from a single or a few lesions to several and/or bulky lesions (surgical resection of a limited disease is the curative approach, but treatment can be more difficult when the interval between new lesions is short, when numerous and bulky metastases are present and multiple treatment modalities have already been performed without results).

The currently available techniques to treat regional IT-mets include:

1. Isolated limb perfusion and isolated limb infusion (Fig. 5.2.4):
   - When melanoma IT-mets are confined to the extremities, the isolation of the affected limb from the systemic circulation represents an opportunity for such a therapeutic approach.
   - Isolation can be achieved by surgical access to the artery and vein on iliac, femoral, popliteal, axillary, or brachial level. The artery and

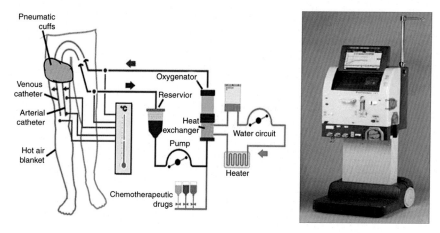

FIGURE 5.2.4 **Regional perfusion.**

vein are clamped and cannulated after which the catheters can be connected to a heart–lung machine to get an oxygenated circuit. To further isolate the limb, a tourniquet is placed proximal to the site of perfusion.

3.2 Isolated Limb Perfusion

- It achieves a 20-fold concentration of chemotherapeutic drugs when compared with systemic therapy [70–72].
- Melphalan (L-phenylalanine mustard) has been the standard drug used in ILP because of its efficacy and toxicity profile [73].
- Standard dosages: 10 mg/L for lower limbs and 13 mg/L for upper limbs.
- The major risk related to ILP is the potential leakage of the effective agents to the systemic circulation; therefore a careful leakage monitoring is mandatory.
- Since the introduction of ILP, some variables, such as temperature, drugs, and procedure indications have been analyzed to improve tumor response.
- The temperature of the skin has to be warmed during perfusion to prevent vasoconstriction in the dermal and epidermal tissues: especially in superficial IT-mets, application of a warm water mattress can improve local drug delivery (the uptake of the drug by IT-mets in vivo is twice as high at 39.5°C than at 37°C [74], and hyperthermia improves the uptake in tumor cells, especially at temperatures greater than 41°C [75,76]). However, tissue temperatures of 41.5–43°C during ILP can yield high response rates [77], but the local toxicity of these

procedures can lead to severe complications [78]. *Mild hyperthermia for ILP is employed as a safer compromise between effectiveness of response and risk of high toxicity.*

Tumor necrosis factor-alpha (TNF-α) was introduced in association with melphalan to improve the action of ILP [79]. TNF has a dual mechanism of action: the direct cytotoxic effect on high-dose TNF to tumor cells [80] and the effect that induces a hemorrhagic necrosis on tumor cells [81]. While the systemic employment of this cytokine must be carefully managed because of its important side effects [82], *in the ILP the advantage of the TNF antitumor activity, in the absence of systemic effects, is increased in hyperthermic conditions with the addition of alkylating agents* [83–85] (the dose of TNF of 1 mg for the arm and 2 mg for the leg is as effective as the higher doses) [86–89].

3.3 Isolated Limb Infusion

It was described by Thompson et al. as a simplified alternative to ILP [90]. Percutaneous arterial and venous catheters are placed in the affected extremity and a tourniquet is placed proximal to the catheter tips to allow isolation of the limb from the systemic circulation.

High dose of a cytotoxic combination of melphalan and actinomycin D is generally used; drugs are infused into a hyperthermic, limb via the arterial catheter and blood is withdrawn from the venous catheter to be reinfused into the arterial side. Drug circulation time is 20–30 min under mild hyperthermic conditions of 38–39°C. ILI is a quicker and safer procedure with response rates similar to those of ILP [91].

- Despite ILP and ILI achieving excellent responses in melanoma IT-mets, the aggressive biological behavior of melanoma determines frequent local recurrent disease in the limbs.
- Reported recurrence rates after perfusion are approximately 50%. Management of residual disease or of disease recurrence following ILP or ILI may include local treatment (by excision) of the remaining or recurrent lesions or ECT as an effective alternative technique to control local disease.
- ILP and ILI can be repeated in selected patients, with results comparable to those obtained using the same techniques at first approach [92,93].
- In consideration of the likelihood of extraregional spread of metastatic cells, patients with IT-mets from melanoma have generally a poor prognosis.
- The duration of survival after these locoregional events seems to be related to the effectiveness of the responses achieved by ILP or ILI; a complete response after these treatments was associated with a median survival of 53 and 44 months, respectively [94,95].

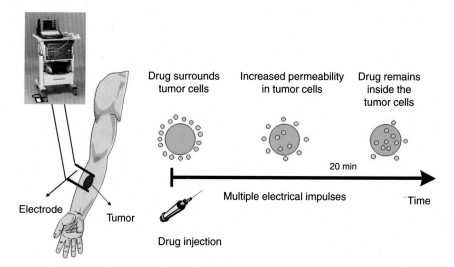

FIGURE 5.2.5 **Electrochemotherapy (ECT).**

- Consequently, a therapeutic approach with these techniques may be considered for subgroups of patients associated with a more favorable tumor biological behavior.

3.4 Electrochemotherapy (Fig. 5.2.5)

- It is an effective therapeutic option for treating melanoma cutaneous and subcutaneous metastases to achieve local tumor control and to preserve the patient's quality of life [96–108].
- The chemotherapeutic agent currently employed is bleomycin (15,000 units/m^2 i.v. in a bolus followed, within 8 min after intravenous injection, by the application of brief electric pulses to each tumor nodule).
- The main eligibility criteria are as follows:
  - Melanoma stage IIIB–C or IV (M1a) [1]
  - Lesions generally not deeper than 3 cm
  - No anticancer treatment 4 weeks before or 8 weeks after ECT treatment
  - Age ≥18 years
  - Eastern Cooperative Oncology Group (ECOG) performance status ≤2
- The main exclusion criteria include:
  - Allergy to bleomycin
  - Severe concomitant disease
  - Life expectancy less than 3 months

- - Active infections
  - Cardiac pacemaker
- Electric current is delivered by means of a 2- to 3-cm long needle electrode, according to lesion size. The electrodes are connected to a pulse generator that produces high voltages (up to 1000 V), but delivered as a compressed train of eight pulses at the frequency of 5000 Hz and 100 μs duration, and are well tolerated by patients.
- ECT could be repeated every 8–12 weeks according to local response, the appearance of new lesions, and patients' compliance to treatment.
- ECT induces a reduction in blood flow within the treated area for up to 24 h, thus leading to tumor hypoxia that causes tumor cell destruction [109,110].
- ECT-induced tumor necrosis stimulates the release of tumor antigens, leading to a local inflammatory and immune reaction [111].
  - ECT represents an effective treatment option for intermediate–advanced stage melanoma patients with cutaneous and subcutaneous metastatic lesions.

3.5 Locoregional Treatments and Systemic Targeted Therapies

- Patients submitted to radical lymph node dissection, to ILP, ILI, or ECT, despite the excellent locoregional results, still have low survival rates. Moreover, these treatments are often associated with relevant side effects.
- In those cases where (poor) prognosis is generally determined by the disease biology, their employment is debated.
- The perspectives have significantly changed after the introduction of BRAF/NRAS/MEK inhibitors, anticytotoxic T-lymphocyte–associated (CTLA) protein-4 antibodies, and PD-1 pathway inhibitors.
- Most patients for whom these new molecules are employed have a stage IV disease, but an increasing number of trials are focusing on patients with unresectable stage III disease; in similar cases, the combination of two different drug delivery methods (systemic and isolated circuit) may represent a logical approach.
  - In conclusion, patients with extensive unresectable IT-mets, associated with an unfavorable survival, should be considered for an integrated therapeutic approach including ILP, ILI, or ECT plus targeted systemic agents.

3.6 Medical Therapy

- In stage III disease, in cases with many IT-mets or satellite metastases, or in cases of relapse notwithstanding repeated surgery, and when the latter is no longer feasible, there is the need for innovative treatment options that may prevent or retard progression from stage III to stage IV (where recently approved systemic treatment options may be adequately employed).

- Intratumoral application of drugs is an appealing therapeutic concept, as high concentrations can be achieved within the tumor with lower systemic toxicity.
- Several cytokines have been used for intratumoral therapy with varying results [112–115].
  - IL-2 intratumoral treatment led to high rate of complete responses and, furthermore, showed an unexpectedly high 5-year OS rate of 61% for stage IIIB/C patients and 38% for stage IV patients [116,117].
  - Used as an intratumoral agent, TNF-α showed local antitumor activity [118].
- L19IL2 and L19TNF are clinical-stage immunocytokines, recombinant human fusion proteins comprising the cytokines IL-2 or TNF, fused to the monoclonal L19 antibody.
- The L19 antibody is a fully human antibody, capable of preferential localization around tumor blood vessels while sparing normal tissues [119,120]. L19, derived from a phage display library of human antibody fragments in the single-chain Fv (scFv) format, recognizes the alternatively spliced extra domain B (EDB) of fibronectin (FN), one of the best characterized markers of angiogenesis [119,121–124].
- L19IL2 is a recombinant fusion protein composed of two portions: L19 and IL-2.
  - L19IL2 has been already studied in advanced solid tumors (renal cell carcinoma [125] and pancreatic cancer).
  - Two studies aimed at assessing the antitumoral activity of systemic L19IL2 administration in combination with DTIC in patients with advanced metastatic melanoma have been carried out, as well as two other clinical trials aimed at assessing the intratumoral effect of L19IL2 either alone or in combination with L19TNF-α in patients suffering from stage III/IV M1a melanoma. These studies confirmed that L19IL2 can be safely and regularly administered to patients with metastatic melanoma.
  - The intralesional treatment of melanoma metastases with L19IL2 (up to 10 MioIU/week for 4 consecutive weeks) in stage III patients resulted in objective responses in about 50% of the lesions [126].
  - The treatment was generally well tolerated. Toxicities were usually mild, of short duration, and limited to inflammatory injection site reaction (local swelling and erythema) in most of treated patients.

- L19TNF is a recombinant fusion protein composed of two portions: L19 and TNF-α.
  - This product has been studied in two different clinical trials:
    - A phase I/II monotherapy study in patients with advanced solid tumors. The main conclusion from this study was that L19TNF can be administered to patients with advanced progressive solid tumors in an outpatient setting up to doses of 13 μg/kg. The observed toxicity profile was mild and reversible [127].
    - A phase I trial in combination with melphalan in the ILP setting for the treatment of patients with metastatic melanoma lesions of the leg, who were candidates for amputation. Five patients were treated with 325 μg and 10 patients with 650 μg of L19TNF. The observed side effects of the L19TNF ILP procedure mainly consisted of reversible and manageable toxicities. Objective responses were observed in the majority of lesions (including some complete responses) while disease progressed outside the perfused limb, as expected. Some examples are shown in Fig. 5.2.4. According to the results of this study, L19TNF can be administered in combination with melphalan and mild hyperthermia, at a dose of 650 μg, in patients with inoperable melanoma lesions of one leg [128].
- Recently, phase III trials have been designed to demonstrate the efficacy of intratumoral administration of L19IL2 + L19TNF followed by surgery in patients suffering from stage IIIB and IIIC metastatic melanoma, as compared to that of surgery alone, in improving RFS.
  - Weekly intratumoral administration of a mixture of 10 MioIU L19IL2 in combination with 312 μg of L19TNF for 4 consecutive weeks into injectable cutaneous/subcutaneous metastases is well tolerated, with few and generally mild recorded adverse events, and is associated with a high proportion of objective responses.
  - Taken together, the benefits of intratumorally administered L19IL2 + L19TNF followed by surgery in terms of local tumor control and improvement of relapse-free survival and OS far outweigh the potential risks that are associated with such a treatment.

References

[1] Balch CM, Gershenwald JE, Soong SJ, et al. Final version of 2009 AJCC melanoma staging and classification. J Clin Oncol 2009;27(36):6199–206.

[2] Balch CM, Gershenwald JE, Soong SJ, et al. Multivariate analysis of prognostic factors among 2,313 patients with stage III melanoma: comparison of nodal micrometastases versus macrometastases. J Clin Oncol 2010;28(14):2452–9.

[3] Gershenwald JE, Ross MI. Sentinel-lymph-node biopsy for cutaneous melanoma. N Engl J Med 2011;364(18):1738–45.

[4] Ross MI, Thompson JF, Gershenwald JE. Sentinel lymph node biopsy for melanoma: critical assessment at its twentieth anniversary. Surg Oncol Clin N Am 2011;20(1):57–78.

[5] Balch CM, Morton DL, Gershenwald JE, et al. Sentinel node biopsy and standard of care for melanoma. J Am Acad Dermatol 2009;60(5):872–5.

[6] Valsecchi ME, Silbermins D, de Rosa N, Wong SL, Lyman GH. Lymphatic mapping and sentinel lymph node biopsy in patients with melanoma: a meta-analysis. J Clin Oncol 2011;29(11):1479–87.

[7] Wrightson WR, Wong SL, Edwards MJ, et al. Complications associated with sentinel lymph node biopsy for melanoma. Ann Surg Oncol 2003;10(6):676–80.

[8] Sondak VK, Taylor JM, Sabel MS, et al. Mitotic rate and younger age are predictors of sentinel lymph node positivity: lessons learned from the generation of a probabilistic model. Ann Surg Oncol 2004;11(3):247–58.

[9] Sabel MS, Rice JD, Griffith KA, et al. Validation of statistical predictive models meant to select melanoma patients for sentinel lymph node biopsy. Ann Surg Oncol 2012;19(1):287–93.

[10] Morton DL, Cochran AJ, Thompson JF, et al. Sentinel node biopsy for early-stage melanoma: accuracy and morbidity in MSLT-I, an international multicenter trial. Ann Surg 2005;242(3):302–11. [discussion 11–3].

[11] Morton DL, Thompson JF, Cochran AJ, et al. Final trial report of sentinel-node biopsy versus nodal observation in melanoma. N Engl J Med 2014;370(7):599–609.

[12] McMasters KM, Noyes RD, Reintgen DS, et al. Lessons learned from the Sunbelt Melanoma Trial. J Surg Oncol 2004;86(4):212–23.

[13] van der Ploeg AP, van Akkooi AC, Haydu LE, et al. The prognostic significance of sentinel node tumour burden in melanoma patients: an international, multicenter study of 1539 sentinel node-positive melanoma patients. Eur J Cancer 2014;50(1):111–20.

[14] Leung AM, Morton DL, Ozao-Choy J, et al. Staging of regional lymph nodes in melanoma: a case for including nonsentinel lymph node positivity in the American Joint Committee on Cancer staging system. JAMA Surg 2013;148(9):879–84.

[15] Faries MB, Thompson JF, Cochran A, et al. The impact on morbidity and length of stay of early versus delayed complete lymphadenectomy in melanoma: results of the Multicenter Selective Lymphadenectomy Trial (I). Ann Surg Oncol 2010;17(12):3324–9.

[16] Morton DL, Thompson JF, Cochran AJ, et al. Sentinel-node biopsy or nodal observation in melanoma. N Engl J Med 2006;355(13):1307–17.

[17] Morton DL. Overview and update of the phase III Multicenter Selective Lymphadenectomy Trials (MSLT-I and MSLT-II) in melanoma. Clin Exp Metastasis 2012;29(7):699–706.

[18] Ascierto PA, Gogas HJ, Grob JJ, et al. Adjuvant interferon alfa in malignant melanoma: an interdisciplinary and multinational expert review. Crit Rev Oncol Hematol 2013;85(2):149–61.

[19] Rossi CR, Mozzillo N, Maurichi A, et al. Number of excised lymph nodes as a quality assurance measure for lymphadenectomy in melanoma. JAMA Surg 2014;149(7):700–6.

[20] van Akkooi AC, de Wilt JH, Verhoef C, et al. Clinical relevance of melanoma micrometastases (<0.1 mm) in sentinel nodes: are these nodes to be considered negative? Ann Oncol 2006;17(10):1578–85.

[21] van Akkooi AC, Nowecki ZI, Voit C, et al. Sentinel node tumor burden according to the Rotterdam criteria is the most important prognostic factor for survival in melanoma patients: a multicenter study in 388 patients with positive sentinel nodes. Ann Surg 2008;248(6):949–55.

[22] van Akkooi AC, Verhoef C, Eggermont AM. Importance of tumor load in the sentinel node in melanoma: clinical dilemmas. Nat Rev Clin Oncol 2010;7(8):446–54.

[23] van der Ploeg AP, van Akkooi AC, Rutkowski P, et al. Prognosis in patients with sentinel node-positive melanoma is accurately defined by the combined Rotterdam tumor load and Dewar topography criteria. J Clin Oncol 2011;29(16):2206–14.

[24] Wong SL, Balch CM, Hurley P, et al. Sentinel lymph node biopsy for melanoma: American Society of Clinical Oncology and Society of Surgical Oncology joint clinical practice guideline. J Clin Oncol 2012;30(23):2912–8.

[25] Wong SL, Balch CM, Hurley P, et al. Sentinel lymph node biopsy for melanoma: American Society of Clinical Oncology and Society of Surgical Oncology joint clinical practice guideline. Ann Surg Oncol 2012;19(11):3313–24.
[26] Leiter U, Meier F, Schittek B, Garbe C. The natural course of cutaneous melanoma. J Surg Oncol 2004;86(4):172–8.
[27] Dummer R, Mangana J. Long-term pegylated interferon-alpha and its potential in the treatment of melanoma. Biologics 2009;3:169–82.
[28] Wang W, Edington HD, Rao UN, et al. Modulation of signal transducers and activators of transcription 1 and 3 signaling in melanoma by high-dose IFNalpha2b. Clin Cancer Res 2007;13(5):1523–31.
[29] Hervas-Stubbs S, Perez-Gracia JL, Rouzaut A, Sanmamed MF, Le Bon A, Melero I. Direct effects of type I interferons on cells of the immune system. Clin Cancer Res 2011;17(9):2619–27.
[30] Wheatley K, Ives N, Hancock B, Gore M, Eggermont A, Suciu S. Does adjuvant interferon-alpha for high-risk melanoma provide a worthwhile benefit? A meta-analysis of the randomised trials. Cancer Treat Rev 2003;29(4):241–52.
[31] Wheatley K, Ives N, Eggermont A, et al. Interferon-{alpha} as adjuvant therapy for melanoma: an individual patient data meta-analysis of randomised trials. ASCO annual meeting proceedings. J Clin Oncol 2007;25:8526.
[32] Mocellin S, Pasquali S, Rossi CR, Nitti D. Interferon alpha adjuvant therapy in patients with high-risk melanoma: a systematic review and meta-analysis. J Natl Cancer Inst 2010;102(7):493–501.
[33] Eggermont AM, Suciu S, Santinami M, et al. Adjuvant therapy with pegylated interferon alfa-2b versus observation alone in resected stage III melanoma: final results of EORTC 18991, a randomised phase III trial. Lancet 2008;372(9633):117–26.
[34] Eggermont AM, Suciu S, MacKie R, et al. Post-surgery adjuvant therapy with intermediate doses of interferon alfa 2b versus observation in patients with stage IIb/III melanoma (EORTC 18952): randomised controlled trial. Lancet 2005;366(9492):1189–96.
[35] Flaherty LE, Moon J, Atkins MB, et al. Phase III trial of high-dose interferon alpha-2b versus cisplatin, vinblastine, DTIC plus IL-2 and interferon in patients with high-risk melanoma (SWOG S0008): an intergroup study of CALGB, COG, ECOG, and SWOG. ASCO annual meeting. J Clin Oncol 2012;30.
[36] Finn OJ. Cancer immunology. N Engl J Med 2008;358(25):2704–15.
[37] Van den Eynde BJ, van der Bruggen P. T cell defined tumor antigens. Curr Opin Immunol 1997;9(5):684–93.
[38] De Plaen E, Arden K, Traversari C, et al. Structure, chromosomal localization, and expression of 12 genes of the MAGE family. Immunogenetics 1994;40(5):360–9.
[39] Jungbluth AA, Silva WA Jr, Iversen K, et al. Expression of cancer-testis (CT) antigens in placenta. Cancer Immun 2007;7:15.
[40] Marchand M, Punt CJ, Aamdal S, et al. Immunisation of metastatic cancer patients with MAGE-3 protein combined with adjuvant SBAS-2: a clinical report. Eur J Cancer 2003;39(1):70–7.
[41] Kruit WH, van Ojik HH, Brichard VG, et al. Phase 1/2 study of subcutaneous and intradermal immunization with a recombinant MAGE-3 protein in patients with detectable metastatic melanoma. Int J Cancer 2005;117(4):596–604.
[42] Hocker TL, Singh MK, Tsao H. Melanoma genetics and therapeutic approaches in the 21st century: moving from the benchside to the bedside. J Invest Dermatol 2008;128(11):2575–95.
[43] Davies H, Bignell GR, Cox C, et al. Mutations of the BRAF gene in human cancer. Nature 2002;417(6892):949–54.
[44] Curtin JA, Fridlyand J, Kageshita T, et al. Distinct sets of genetic alterations in melanoma. N Engl J Med 2005;353(20):2135–47.

[45] Garrido MC, Bastian BC. KIT as a therapeutic target in melanoma. J Invest Dermatol 2010;130(1):20–7.

[46] Kumar R, Angelini S, Snellman E, Hemminki K. BRAF mutations are common somatic events in melanocytic nevi. J Invest Dermatol 2004;122(2):342–8.

[47] Gorden A, Osman I, Gai W, et al. Analysis of BRAF and N-RAS mutations in metastatic melanoma tissues. Cancer Res 2003;63(14):3955–7.

[48] Edlundh-Rose E, Egyhazi S, Omholt K, et al. NRAS and BRAF mutations in melanoma tumours in relation to clinical characteristics: a study based on mutation screening by pyrosequencing. Melanoma Res 2006;16(6):471–8.

[49] Goel VK, Lazar AJ, Warneke CL, Redston MS, Haluska FG. Examination of mutations in BRAF, NRAS, and PTEN in primary cutaneous melanoma. J Invest Dermatol 2006;126(1):154–60.

[50] Swaika A, Crozier JA, Joseph RW. Vemurafenib: an evidence-based review of its clinical utility in the treatment of metastatic melanoma. Drug Des Devel Ther 2014;8:775–87.

[51] GlaxoSmithKline. Highlights of prescribing information of Tafinlar (dabrafenib capsules). Brentford, UK: GlaxoSmithKline; 2014.

[52] GlaxoSmithKline. Two new GSK oral oncology treatments, BRAF-inhibitor Tafinlar (dabrafenib) capsules and the first MEK-inhibitor Mekinist (trametinib) tablets, approved by FDA as single-agent therapies. Brentford, UK: GlaxoSmithKline; 2014.

[53] Chapman PB, Hauschild A, Robert C, et al. Improved survival with vemurafenib in melanoma with BRAF V600E mutation. N Engl J Med 2011;364(26):2507–16.

[54] Hauschild A, Grob JJ, Demidov LV, et al. Dabrafenib in BRAF-mutated metastatic melanoma: a multicentre, open-label, phase 3 randomised controlled trial. Lancet 2012;380(9839):358–65.

[55] Flaherty KT, Robert C, Hersey P, et al. Improved survival with MEK inhibition in BRAF-mutated melanoma. N Engl J Med 2012;367(2):107–14.

[56] Flaherty KT, Infante JR, Daud A, et al. Combined BRAF and MEK inhibition in melanoma with BRAF V600 mutations. N Engl J Med 2012;367(18):1694–703.

[57] Hodi FS, O'Day SJ, McDermott DF, et al. Improved survival with ipilimumab in patients with metastatic melanoma. N Engl J Med 2010;363(8):711–23.

[58] Robert C, Thomas L, Bondarenko I, et al. Ipilimumab plus dacarbazine for previously untreated metastatic melanoma. N Engl J Med 2011;364(26):2517–26.

[59] Lebbé C, Weber JS, Maio M, Neyns B, Harmankaya K. Long-term survival in patients with metastatic melanoma who received ipilimumab in four phase II trials. ASCO Annual Meeting. J Clin Oncol 2013;31.

[60] Greenwald RJ, Freeman GJ, Sharpe AH. The B7 family revisited. Annu Rev Immunol 2005;23:515–48.

[61] Okazaki T, Maeda A, Nishimura H, Kurosaki T, Honjo T. PD-1 immunoreceptor inhibits B cell receptor-mediated signaling by recruiting src homology 2-domain-containing tyrosine phosphatase 2 to phosphotyrosine. Proc Natl Acad Sci USA 2001;98(24):13866–71.

[62] Topalian SL, Hodi FS, Brahmer JR, et al. Safety, activity, and immune correlates of anti-PD-1 antibody in cancer. N Engl J Med 2012;366(26):2443–54.

[63] Sznol M, Kluger HM, Hodi FS, et al. Survival and long-term follow-up of safety and response in patients (pts) with advanced melanoma (MEL) in a phase I trial of nivolumab (anti-PD-1; BMS-936558; ONO-4538). J Clin Oncol 2013;31.

[64] Hamid O, Robert C, Daud A, et al. Safety and tumor responses with lambrolizumab (anti-PD-1) in melanoma. N Engl J Med 2013;369(2):134–44.

[65] Thompson RH, Dong H, Lohse CM, et al. PD-1 is expressed by tumor-infiltrating immune cells and is associated with poor outcome for patients with renal cell carcinoma. Clin Cancer Res 2007;13(6):1757–61.

[66] Nomi T, Sho M, Akahori T, et al. Clinical significance and therapeutic potential of the programmed death-1 ligand/programmed death-1 pathway in human pancreatic cancer. Clin Cancer Res 2007;13(7):2151–7.

[67] Gao Q, Wang XY, Qiu SJ, et al. Overexpression of PD-L1 significantly associates with tumor aggressiveness and postoperative recurrence in human hepatocellular carcinoma. Clin Cancer Res 2009;15(3):971–9.

[68] Hamanishi J, Mandai M, Iwasaki M, et al. Programmed cell death 1 ligand 1 and tumor-infiltrating CD8+ T lymphocytes are prognostic factors of human ovarian cancer. Proc Natl Acad Sci USA 2007;104(9):3360–5.

[69] Robert C, Schachter J, Long GV, et al. Pembrolizumab versus ipilimumab in advanced melanoma. N Engl J Med 2015;372(26):2521–32.

[70] Creech O Jr, Krementz ET, Ryan RF, Winblad JN. Chemotherapy of cancer: regional perfusion utilizing an extracorporeal circuit. Ann Surg 1958;148(4):616–32.

[71] Benckhuijsen C, Kroon BB, van Geel AN, Wieberdink J. Regional perfusion treatment with melphalan for melanoma in a limb: an evaluation of drug kinetics. Eur J Surg Oncol 1988;14(2):157–63.

[72] Vrouenraets BC, Nieweg OE, Kroon BB. Thirty-five years of isolated limb perfusion for melanoma: indications and results. Br J Surg 1996;83(10):1319–28.

[73] Thompson JF, Gianoutsos MP. Isolated limb perfusion for melanoma: effectiveness and toxicity of cisplatin compared with that of melphalan and other drugs. World J Surg 1992;16(2):227–33.

[74] Omlor G. Optimization of isolated hyperthermic limb perfusion. World J Surg 1993;17(1):134.

[75] Cavaliere R, Ciocatto EC, Giovanella BC, et al. Selective heat sensitivity of cancer cells. Biochemical and clinical studies. Cancer 1967;20(9):1351–81.

[76] Clark J, Grabs AJ, Parsons PG, Smithers BM, Addison RS, Roberts MS. Melphalan uptake, hyperthermic synergism and drug resistance in a human cell culture model for the isolated limb perfusion of melanoma. Melanoma Res 1994;4(6):365–70.

[77] Di Filippo F, Anza M, Rossi CR, et al. The application of hyperthermia in regional chemotherapy. Semin Surg Oncol 1998;14(3):215–23.

[78] Kroon BB, Klaase JM, van Geel AN. Application of hyperthermia in regional isolated perfusion for melanoma of the limbs. Reg Cancer Treat 1992;4:223–6.

[79] Carswell EA, Old LJ, Kassel RL, Green S, Fiore N, Williamson B. An endotoxin-induced serum factor that causes necrosis of tumors. Proc Natl Acad Sci USA 1975;72(9):3666–70.

[80] Sugarman BJ, Aggarwal BB, Hass PE, Figari IS, Palladino MA Jr, Shepard HM. Recombinant human tumor necrosis factor-alpha: effects on proliferation of normal and transformed cells in vitro. Science 1985;230(4728):943–5.

[81] Watanabe N, Niitsu Y, Umeno H, et al. Toxic effect of tumor necrosis factor on tumor vasculature in mice. Cancer Res 1988;48(8):2179–83.

[82] Feldman ER, Creagan ET, Schaid DJ, Ahmann DL. Phase II trial of recombinant tumor necrosis factor in disseminated malignant melanoma. Am J Clin Oncol 1992;15(3):256–9.

[83] Watanabe N, Niitsu Y, Umeno H, et al. Synergistic cytotoxic and antitumor effects of recombinant human tumor necrosis factor and hyperthermia. Cancer Res 1988;48(3):650–3.

[84] Regenass U, Muller M, Curschellas E, Matter A. Anti-tumor effects of tumor necrosis factor in combination with chemotherapeutic agents. Int J Cancer 1987;39(2):266–73.

[85] Lienard D, Ewalenko P, Delmotte JJ, Renard N, Lejeune FJ. High-dose recombinant tumor necrosis factor alpha in combination with interferon gamma and melphalan in isolation perfusion of the limbs for melanoma and sarcoma. J Clin Oncol 1992;10(1):52–60.

[86] de Wilt JH, Manusama ER, van Tiel ST, van Ijken MG, ten Hagen TL, Eggermont AM. Prerequisites for effective isolated limb perfusion using tumour necrosis factor alpha and melphalan in rats. Br J Cancer 1999;80(1-2):161–6.

[87] Bonvalot S, Laplanche A, Lejeune F, et al. Limb salvage with isolated perfusion for soft tissue sarcoma: could less TNF-alpha be better? Ann Oncol 2005;16(7):1061–8.

[88] Hill S, Fawcett WJ, Sheldon J, Soni N, Williams T, Thomas JM. Low-dose tumour necrosis factor alpha and melphalan in hyperthermic isolated limb perfusion. Br J Surg 1993;80(8):995–7.

[89] Rossi CR, Foletto M, Mocellin S, Pilati P, Lise M. Hyperthermic isolated limb perfusion with low-dose tumor necrosis factor-alpha and melphalan for bulky in-transit melanoma metastases. Ann Surg Oncol 2004;11(2):173–7.

[90] Thompson JF, Waugh RC, Schacherer CW. Isolated limb infusion with melphalan for recurrent limb melanoma: a simple alternative to isolated limb perfusion. Reg Cancer Treat 1994;7:188–92.

[91] Kroon HM, Moncrieff M, Kam PC, Thompson JF. Factors predictive of acute regional toxicity after isolated limb infusion with melphalan and actinomycin D in melanoma patients. Ann Surg Oncol 2009;16(5):1184–92.

[92] Grunhagen DJ, van Etten B, Brunstein F, et al. Efficacy of repeat isolated limb perfusions with tumor necrosis factor alpha and melphalan for multiple in-transit metastases in patients with prior isolated limb perfusion failure. Ann Surg Oncol 2005;12(8):609–15.

[93] Kroon HM, Lin DY, Kam PC, Thompson JF. Efficacy of repeat isolated limb infusion with melphalan and actinomycin D for recurrent melanoma. Cancer 2009;115(9):1932–40.

[94] Deroose JP, Eggermont AM, van Geel AN, de Wilt JH, Burger JW, Verhoef C. 20 years experience of TNF-based isolated limb perfusion for in-transit melanoma metastases: TNF dose matters. Ann Surg Oncol 2012;19(2):627–35.

[95] Kroon HM, Moncrieff M, Kam PC, Thompson JF. Outcomes following isolated limb infusion for melanoma. A 14-year experience. Ann Surg Oncol 2008;15(11):3003–13.

[96] Belehradek M, Domenge C, Luboinski B, Orlowski S, Belehradek J Jr, Mir LM. Electrochemotherapy, a new antitumor treatment. First clinical phase I–II trial. Cancer 1993;72(12):3694–700.

[97] Mir LM, Orlowski S. Mechanisms of electrochemotherapy. Adv Drug Deliv Rev 1999;35(1):107–18.

[98] Mir LM, Glass LF, Sersa G, et al. Effective treatment of cutaneous and subcutaneous malignant tumours by electrochemotherapy. Br J Cancer 1998;77(12):2336–42.

[99] Rols MP, Bachaud JM, Giraud P, Chevreau C, Roche H, Teissie J. Electrochemotherapy of cutaneous metastases in malignant melanoma. Melanoma Res 2000;10(5):468–74.

[100] Byrne CM, Thompson JF, Johnston H, et al. Treatment of metastatic melanoma using electroporation therapy with bleomycin (electrochemotherapy). Melanoma Res 2005;15(1):45–51.

[101] Gaudy C, Richard MA, Folchetti G, Bonerandi JJ, Grob JJ. Randomized controlled study of electrochemotherapy in the local treatment of skin metastases of melanoma. J Cutan Med Surg 2006;10(3):115–21.

[102] Larkin JO, Collins CG, Aarons S, et al. Electrochemotherapy: aspects of preclinical development and early clinical experience. Ann Surg 2007;245(3):469–79.

[103] Sersa G, Stabuc B, Cemazar M, Miklavcic D, Rudolf Z. Electrochemotherapy with cisplatin: the systemic antitumour effectiveness of cisplatin can be potentiated locally by the application of electric pulses in the treatment of malignant melanoma skin metastases. Melanoma Res 2000;10(4):381–5.

[104] Domenge C, Orlowski S, Luboinski B, et al. Antitumor electrochemotherapy: new advances in the clinical protocol. Cancer 1996;77(5):956–63.

[105] Campana LG, Mocellin S, Basso M, et al. Bleomycin-based electrochemotherapy: clinical outcome from a single institution's experience with 52 patients. Ann Surg Oncol 2009;16(1):191–9.

[106] Kis E, Olah J, Ocsai H, et al. Electrochemotherapy of cutaneous metastases of melanoma—a case series study and systematic review of the evidence. Dermatol Surg 2011;37(6):816–24.

[107] Marty M, Sersa G, Garbay JR, et al. Electrochemotherapy—an easy, highly effective and safe treatment of cutaneous and subcutaneous metastases: results of ESOPE study. Eur J Cancer Suppl 2006;4:3–13.

[108] Mir LM, Gehl J, Sersa G, et al. Standard operating procedures of the electrochemotherapy: instructions for the use of bleomycin or cisplatin administered either systemically

or locally and electric pulses delivered by the Cliniporator by means of invasive or non-invasive electrodes. Eur J Cancer Suppl 2006;4:14–25.

[109] Markelc B, Sersa G, Cemazar M. Differential mechanisms associated with vascular disrupting action of electrochemotherapy: intravital microscopy on the level of single normal and tumor blood vessels. PLoS One 2013;8(3):e59557.

[110] Sersa G, Jarm T, Kotnik T, et al. Vascular disrupting action of electroporation and electrochemotherapy with bleomycin in murine sarcoma. Br J Cancer 2008;98(2):388–98.

[111] Reinhold U. Electrochemotherapy of skin tumors. Hautarzt 2011;62(7):549–58. [quiz 59].

[112] Cornejo P, Vanaclocha F, Polimon I, Del Rio R. Intralesional interferon treatment of lentigo maligna. Arch Dermatol 2000;136(3):428–30.

[113] Vaquerano JE, Cadbury P, Treseler P, Sagebiel R, Leong SP. Regression of in-transit melanoma of the scalp with intralesional recombinant human granulocyte-macrophage colony-stimulating factor. Arch Dermatol 1999;135(10):1276–7.

[114] von Wussow P, Block B, Hartmann F, Deicher H. Intralesional interferon-alpha therapy in advanced malignant melanoma. Cancer 1988;61(6):1071–4.

[115] Gutwald J, Groth W, Mahrle G. Peritumoral administered IL-2-induced tumor regression in melanoma. Pilot study. Hautarzt 1994;45(8):536–40.

[116] Radny P, Caroli UM, Bauer J, et al. Phase II trial of intralesional therapy with interleukin-2 in soft-tissue melanoma metastases. Br J Cancer 2003;89(9):1620–6.

[117] Weide B, Derhovanessian E, Pflugfelder A, et al. High response rate after intratumoral treatment with interleukin-2: results from a phase 2 study in 51 patients with metastasized melanoma. Cancer 2010;116(17):4139–46.

[118] Bartsch HH, Pfizenmaier K, Schroeder M, Nagel GA. Intralesional application of recombinant human tumor necrosis factor alpha induces local tumor regression in patients with advanced malignancies. Eur J Cancer Clin Oncol 1989;25(2):287–91.

[119] Neri D, Bicknell R. Tumour vascular targeting. Nat Rev Cancer 2005;5(6):436–46.

[120] Trachsel E, Neri D. Antibodies for angiogenesis inhibition, vascular targeting and endothelial cell transcytosis. Adv Drug Deliv Rev 2006;58(5–6):735–54.

[121] Borsi L, Balza E, Bestagno M, et al. Selective targeting of tumoral vasculature: comparison of different formats of an antibody (L19) to the ED-B domain of fibronectin. Int J Cancer 2002;102(1):75–85.

[122] Carnemolla B, Neri D, Castellani P, et al. Phage antibodies with pan-species recognition of the oncofoetal angiogenesis marker fibronectin ED-B domain. Int J Cancer 1996;68(3):397–405.

[123] Castellani P, Borsi L, Carnemolla B, et al. Differentiation between high- and low-grade astrocytoma using a human recombinant antibody to the extra domain-B of fibronectin. Am J Pathol 2002;161(5):1695–700.

[124] Rybak JN, Trachsel E, Scheuermann J, Neri D. Ligand-based vascular targeting of disease. ChemMedChem 2007;2(1):22–40.

[125] Johannsen M, Spitaleri G, Curigliano G, et al. The tumour-targeting human L19-IL2 immunocytokine: preclinical safety studies, phase I clinical trial in patients with solid tumours and expansion into patients with advanced renal cell carcinoma. Eur J Cancer 2010;46(16):2926–35.

[126] Weide B, Eigentler TK, Pflugfelder A, et al. Intralesional treatment of stage III metastatic melanoma patients with L19-IL2 results in sustained clinical and systemic immunologic responses. Cancer Immunol Res 2014;2(7):668–78.

[127] Spitaleri G, Berardi R, Pierantoni C, et al. Phase I/II study of the tumour-targeting human monoclonal antibody–cytokine fusion protein L19-TNF in patients with advanced solid tumours. J Cancer Res Clin Oncol 2013;139(3):447–55.

[128] Papadia F, Basso V, Patuzzo R, et al. Isolated limb perfusion with the tumor-targeting human monoclonal antibody–cytokine fusion protein L19-TNF plus melphalan and mild hyperthermia in patients with locally advanced extremity melanoma. J Surg Oncol 2013;107(2):173–9.

Further Reading

Wong SL, Morton DL, Thompson JF, et al. Melanoma patients with positive sentinel nodes who did not undergo completion lymphadenectomy: a multi-institutional study. Ann Surg Oncol 2006;13(6):809–16.

Kingham TP, Panageas KS, Ariyan CE, Busam KJ, Brady MS, Coit DG. Outcome of patients with a positive sentinel lymph node who do not undergo completion lymphadenectomy. Ann Surg Oncol 2010;17(2):514–20.

Calabro A, Singletary SE, Balch CM. Patterns of relapse in 1001 consecutive patients with melanoma nodal metastases. Arch Surg 1989;124(9):1051–5.

Grunhagen DJ, de Wilt JH, ten Hagen TL, Eggermont AM. Technology insight: utility of TNF-alpha-based isolated limb perfusion to avoid amputation of irresectable tumors of the extremities. Nat Clin Pract Oncol 2006;3(2):94–103.

Lejeune FJ, Lienard D, Matter M, Ruegg C. Efficiency of recombinant human TNF in human cancer therapy. Cancer Immun 2006;6:6.

Nishimura T, Ohta S, Sato N, Togashi Y, Goto M, Hashimoto Y. Combination tumor-immunotherapy with recombinant tumor necrosis factor and recombinant interleukin 2 in mice. Int J Cancer 1987;40(2):255–61.

Schwager K, Hemmerle T, Aebischer D, Neri D. The immunocytokine L19-IL2 eradicates cancer when used in combination with CTLA-4 blockade or with L19-TNF. J Invest Dermatol 2013;133(3):751–8.

SUBCHAPTER

5.3

The Treatment of Stage IV Metastatic Melanoma

Pietro Quaglino, Paolo Fava, Maria T. Fierro

University of Turin, Turin, Italy

1 PATIENT CHARACTERISTICS, DISEASE EVALUATION, AND TREATMENT OPTIONS

There are some parameters that may correctly drive our evaluation on the best treatment for the patient we are dealing with (Table 5.3.1).

- Clinical scenario examples:
  - If low tumor burden (e.g., one or two localized mets), low progression pattern, and good PS:
    - Local therapies (surgery)
    - Immunotherapy even if BRAF mutated

TABLE 5.3.1   Decision-Making Factors in Advanced Metastatic Melanoma: Pretreatment Parameters to Be Evaluated

Parameter	Significance	Marker
Mutation pattern	• Possibility to prescribe a molecular target therapy	BRAF, NRAS, c-Kit
Performance status (PS)	• Candidate for active therapy or only palliation • Need to obtain a quick response	ECOG
High/low tumor load	• Responsiveness to systemic treatment	LDH Blood chemistry CT/MRI images
Brain mets	• Risk of CNS symptoms	CT/MRI images
Progression pattern (low/fast)	• Responsiveness to systemic treatment • Need to obtain a quick response	LDH CT/MRI images
Clinical trials	• Availability of clinical trials	NA

Modified from an oral communication by Prof. Axel Hauschild at ASCO 2014.

- • If unfavorable PS, high tumor load, fast progression pattern, and brain mets:
    - – Target therapies with anti-BRAF and anti-MEK (if BRAF mutated)
    - – Palliation

- • The main difference in the clinical activity between target therapies and immunotherapy is the early response induction of the target therapies.
- • Both regimens are significantly more active in the presence of a low tumor burden.
- • LDH values are related to:
    - • The turnover of growth of metastatic cells
    - • The reduction of extracellular pH (maybe associated with an impairment of lymphocyte functions)
    - • Unfavorable prognostic factor in patients treated by ipilimumab

The treatment options that can be considered are represented by local and systemic therapies (Table 5.3.2).

Local and systemic approaches need to be integrated in the same patient to obtain the best results (Figs. 5.3.1 and 5.3.2).

TABLE 5.3.2   Treatment Options

Local	Systemic
Surgery	Target therapies • Anti-BRAF (vemurafenib, dabrafenib) • Anti-MEK (trametinib, cobimetinib) • c-Kit inhibitors (imatinib, dasatinib)
Radiotherapy	Immunotherapy (checkpoint inhibitors) • Anti–CTLA-4 (ipilimumab) • Anti–PD-1 (nivolumab, pembrolizumab)
Electrochemotherapy (skin mets)	Chemotherapy • Dacarbazine • Temozolomide • Fotemustine • Integrated polichemotherapy regimens with or without interleukin-2
Thermoablation (mainly liver mets)	

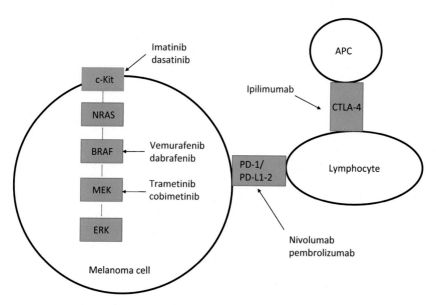

FIGURE 5.3.1   **Immune checkpoint inhibitors and targeted therapies in stage IV metastatic melanoma.**

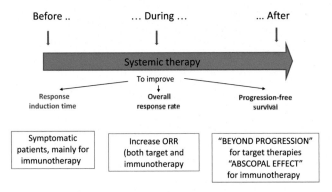

FIGURE 5.3.2 **Association of local and systemic therapies: why, when, and in which patients.**

2 SURGICAL THERAPY

Surgery of stage IV metastatic melanoma still constitutes a relevant therapeutic tool that can be considered to treat a localized disease or a symptomatic lesion in a patient with widespread disease:

- First choice of therapy in about 25% of stage IV patients
- Allows the complete removal of a lesion with acceptable morbidity and mortality
- Selection criteria for patients amenable to surgical treatment:
  - Limited disease extension with the possibility to completely resect the disease burden
  - Previous prolonged disease-free survival
  - Tumor volume doubling time potentially >60 days
- Patients treated by surgery with or without standard medical treatment have a survival advantage versus patients treated by standard medical treatment alone.
- Surgery can be positively associated with immunotherapy in an attempt to reduce the disease burden and thus increase the effectiveness of the immune response and of the treatment.
- Surgery can be favorably associated with target therapy, to increase the percentage of complete responses and thus render the patient no evidence of disease (NED) or to manage the local progression and maintain the systemic treatment ("beyond progression").

3 RADIOTHERAPY

Melanoma is generally considered to be a radioresistant neoplasia; thus radiation therapy has for long time represented only a palliative option for many patients with metastatic melanoma.

Palliation radiotherapy was considered for patients with painful lesions mainly located to the bones, nodes, or skin; in presence of bleeding not amenable with other treatments; or in patients with brain metastases to manage the symptoms related to edema.

- "Whole-brain radiotherapy" (WBRT):
  - For patients with multiple cerebral metastases
  - A total of 30 Gy delivered in 10 fractions during 2 weeks (most common schedule)
  - No significant impact on overall survival
  - Detrimental neurocognitive outcomes
- Stereotactic ablative radiotherapy (SABR):
  - Delivery of highly focused doses in 1 or few sessions (<10), administered with ablative intent
  - Promising progression-free survival
  - Limited toxicity
  - Stereotactic radiosurgery (SRS)—brain or spine:
    - For patients with low number of brain metastases with limited dimensions
    - Alone or in association with targeted therapies or immune therapy
  - Stereotactic body radiation therapy (SBRT): one or several stereotactic radiation treatments within the body, such as the lungs

Today the association between SRS and immune therapy is intriguing:

- Ionizing radiations seems to:
  - Have proinflammatory effects
  - Convert the tumor in an "in situ" vaccine
  - Alter the microenvironment toward the development of an "immunogenic hub"
  - Promote both the priming and effector phases of antitumor immune response
- This phenomenon may explain the well-known "abscopal" effect:
  - Radiotherapy on a new lesion after ipilimumab may induce a response also in preexisting sites not responding to the anti–CTLA-4 treatment.
  - It is occasionally observed in patients undergoing palliative radiotherapy.
  - Most patients were treated for disease progression at a median time of 5 months after the last ipilimumab dose.
  - OS for patients with abscopal response was significantly higher than for patients without abscopal response (22.4 vs. 8.3 months).
- On the contrary, it is not possible to perform radiotherapy during treatment with BRAF inhibitors (BRAFi) due to the potential

occurrence of skin side effects from moderate to severe on the site of radiotherapy or as recall dermatitis.

- Interrupt the treatment with BRAFi for a certain period of time before and after radiotherapy.

4 ELECTROCHEMOTHERAPY

- Therapeutic tool for the local treatment of cutaneous and subcutaneous metastases
- Delivery of electric pulses directly onto the skin lesions in association with the administration, by local or systemic injections, of a low dosage of chemotherapy (bleomycin or cisplatin)
- Response rates ranging up to 90% of treated lesions
- Indicated in patients with locoregional metastases, that is, with stage III melanoma
- In stage IV patients, due to widespread disease, is restricted to selected cases:
  - Can be associated with increase in the local response in the skin or to induce responses in sites not responding to systemic treatment
  - May (as radiotherapy) boost antitumor immunity by promoting Langerhans cell migration and dendritic cell recruitment, thus inducing a sort of "in situ" vaccination

5 MEDICAL THERAPY

Until the recent years, the medical management of metastatic melanoma not treatable by surgery was based on the use of chemotherapy either as single agent (dacarbazine, temozolomide, or fotemustine) or as polichemotherapy with or without biotherapy (e.g., interferon).

The introduction of new drugs (immune checkpoint inhibitors and targeted therapies) completely modified the therapeutic approach and induced an overwhelming improvement in the survival rates of these patients.

5.1 Immune Checkpoint Inhibitors: Anti–CTLA-4

5.1.1 Ipilimumab

- It is a fully humanized monoclonal antibody, which binds to CTLA-4, a receptor expressed on the T-cell surface that interacts with CD80 (B7-1) and CD86 (B7-2) on the antigen-presenting cells (APCs) and downregulates T-cell response.

- CTLA-4 blockade allows CD28 to bind to B7-1 receptors, leading to immune activation, IL-2 secretion, and cytotoxic T-cell upregulation and proliferation.
- The interaction of ipilimumab with the immune system therefore takes place in an early phase of the immune response involving "naive" T lymphocytes and the APCs.
- This mechanism of action explains:
  - The characteristics of the clinical activity (delayed occurrence of a relevant clinical response)
  - The common side effects, consisting of immune-mediated reactions developing more frequently in the skin, gastrointestinal tract (mainly diarrhea), liver, and endocrinal glands (Table 5.3.3; Fig. 5.3.3)

TABLE 5.3.3 More Frequent Adverse Events From Immune Checkpoint Inhibitors (Anti–CTLA-4 and Anti–PD-1) Alone or in Combination and From Targeted Therapies With Anti-BRAF Inhibitors Alone or in Combination With MEK Inhibitors

Drug/regimen	More frequently reported adverse events (%)				
Ipilimumab (Hodi, 2010) [1]	Dermatologic (43%)	Fatigue (42%)	Diarrhea (32.8%)	Nausea, vomiting (23.7%)	Endocrine (7.6%)
Pembrolizumab (KEYNOTE-002) [2]	Fatigue (21%)	Pruritus (21%)	Rash (12%)	Diarrhea (8%)	Arthralgia (7%)
Nivolumab + ipilimumab (Hodi, 2015) [3]	Diarrhea (45%)	Rash (41%)	Fatigue (39%)	Pruritus (35%)	Nausea, liver (22%)
Vemurafenib (BRIM-3) [4]	Rash (49%)	SCC (14%) Papilloma (15%) Hyper-keratosis (19%)	Arthralgia (39%)	Fatigue (34%)	Photosensi-tivity (31%)
Dabrafenib (BREAK-2)	Hyperkeratosis (27%) Papilloma (15%) SCC (10%)	Arthralgia (33%)	Fever (24%%)	Fatigue (22%)	Headache (21%%)
Dabrafenib + trametinib (Combi D) [5]	Fever (51%)	Fatigue (35%)	Headache (30%)	Nausea (30%)	Chills (30%)
Vemurafenib + cobimetinib (CoBrim) [6]	Diarrhea (56%)	Nausea (40%)	Vomiting (21%)	Rash (38%)	Photosensi-tivity (28%)

SCC, Squamous cell carcinoma.

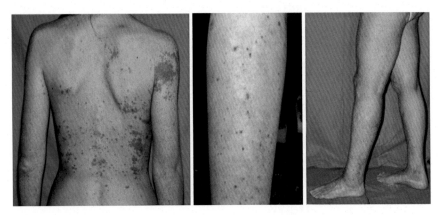

FIGURE 5.3.3 **Cutaneous side effects from ipilimumab.** From left to right: skin rash with erythematous edematous lesions; vasculitis-like lesions on the lower limb; and vitiligo-like lesion on the lower limbs. Clinical expression of an immune activation against melanoma-associated antigens.

- Both 3- and 10-mg/kg dose regimens induce the best response even if the latter dose is coupled with an increase in immune-related adverse effects.
- Ipilimumab alone or in association with different agents has been compared with the same agent in monotherapy (gp100 vaccine/dacarbazine) resulting always in better OS.
- It produces a plateau in survival curves (around 3 years after treatment with follow-up of up to 10 years).
- Three-year OS rates were 22, 26, and 20% for all, treatment-naive, and previously treated patients, respectively.
- Distinct response patterns have been described:
  - Shrinkage in baseline lesions, without new lesions
  - Durable stable disease (in some patients followed by a slow, steady decline in total tumor burden)
  - Response after an increase in total tumor burden:
    - Due to inflammatory changes and the recall of T cells and other immune cells to tumor site
  - Response in the presence of new lesions

Table 5.3.4 summarizes the results of the trials investigating ipilimumab for unresectable or metastatic melanoma.

5.2 Immune Checkpoint Inhibitors: Anti–PD-1/PDL-1

5.2.1 Nivolumab
- A fully human IgG4 anti–PD-1 monoclonal antibody

TABLE 5.3.4 Summary of the Most Relevant Studies on CTLA-4 Inhibitors in Melanoma in Terms of Clinical Activity

Author	Study design	Drug(s)	No. of patients	RR (%)	DCR (%)	OS (median; months)	1-Year % OS	2-Year % OS	3-Year % OS
Wolchok (2010) [7]	Randomized, double blind, phase 2 trial	Ipilimumab10 mg/kg Ipilimumab 3 mg/kg Ipilimumab 0.3 mg/kg	73 72 72	11.1 4.2 0	29.2 26.4 13.7	11.4 8.7 8.6	48.6 39.3 39.6	29.8 24.2 18.4	NA
Hodi (2010) [1]	Randomized, double blind, phase 3	Ipilimumab + gp100 Ipilimumab alone gp100 alone	403 137 136	5.7 10.9 1.5	20.1 28.5 11	10 10.1 6.4	43.6 45.6 25.3%	21.6 23.5 13.7	NA
Robert (2011) [8]	Randomized, double blind, phase 2	Ipilimumab + dacarbazine Dacarbazine + placebo	250 252	15.2 10.3	33.2 30.1	11.2 9.1	47.3 36.3	28.5 17.9	20.8 12.2
Schadendorf (2015) [9]	Pooled analysis	Ipilimumab	1861	—	—	11.4	—	—	22

DCR, Disease control rate; OS, overall survival; RR, response rate.

5.2.2 Pembrolizumab

- A humanized IgG4 anti–PD-1 monoclonal antibody

5.2.3 Mechanism of Action

- PD-1 protein is a coinhibitory receptor expressed on B and T cells, and is involved in the negative regulation of T-cell activation.
- PD-1 ligand (PDL-1) is expressed in different tumors, is associated with a worse prognosis, and its expression and interaction with T cells is thought to be one of the mechanisms underlying immune system escape.
- Nivolumab and pembrolizumab block the interaction between PD-1 and PDL-1.

5.2.4 Efficacy Data

- Nivolumab versus dacarbazine:
  - One-year OS (overall survival): 72.9% versus 42.1%
  - ORR (overall response rate): 40% versus 13.9%
  - AE (adverse events): 11.7% versus 17.6% of patients
- Pembrolizumab, ORR: 38%
- Pembrolizumab, 2 versus 10 mg/kg:
  - ORR: 26% for both
  - PFS (progression free survival): 22 versus 14 weeks
- Pembrolizumab (2 or 10 mg/kg) versus chemotherapy:
  - PFS: 5.4, 5.8 versus 3.6 months
  - AE occurred earlier in patients given chemotherapy
- Pembrolizumab (10 mg/kg every 2 or 3 weeks) versus ipilimumab (four doses—3 mg/kg every 3 weeks):
  - Six-month progression-free survival rates: 47.3, 46.4% versus 26.5%
  - Twelve-month survival rates: 74.1, 68.4% versus 58.2%
  - ORR: 33.7, 32.9% versus 11.9%
  - AE of grade 3–5 severity lower in the pembrolizumab groups (13.3 and 10.1%) than in the ipilimumab group (19.9%)
- The toxicity profile of anti–PD-1 agents resulted similar to that of anti–CTLA-4.
- Table 5.3.5 summarizes the results of the trials investigating nivolumab and pembrolizumab for unresectable or metastatic melanoma.

5.2.5 Association of Anti–CTLA-4 and Anti–PD-1

- Recent data demonstrated an improvement in ORR and OS for the combination of ipilimumab and anti–PD-1 agents but around 50% of patients included in the study experienced grade 3 or 4 treatment-related adverse events.

TABLE 5.3.5 Summary of the Most Relevant Studies on PD-1 Inhibitors Alone or in Combination With Ipilimumab in Melanoma in Terms of Clinical Activity

Author	Study design	Drug(s)	No. of patients	RR (%)	1-year % OS	Median PFS
Robert (2014) [10]	Randomized, double blind, phase 3	Nivolumab Dacarbazine	210 208	40 13.9	72.9 42.1	5.1 months 2.2 months
Robert (2015) [11]	Randomized, double blind, phase 3	Pembrolizumab Q2W Pembrolizumab Q3W Ipilimumab	279 277 278	33.7 32.9 11.9	74.1 68.4 58.2	47.3% 46.4% 26.5% (% 6 months)
Ribas (2015) [2]	Randomized, double blind, phase 2	Pembrolizumab 10 mg/kg Pembrolizumab 2 mg/kg Chemotherapy	181 180 179	— 	— 	5.8 months 5.4 months 3.6 months
Wolchok (2013) [12]	Phase 1	Ipilimumab–nivolumab: • Sequenced treatment • Combined treatment	 33 53	 40 40	 — 	 —
Larkin (2015) [6]	Randomized, double blind, phase 3	Nivolumab + ipilimumab Ipilimumab Nivolumab	314 315 316	57.6 19 43.7	— 	11.5 months 2.9 months 6.9 months
Hodi (2015) [3]	Randomized, double blind, phase 2	Nivolumab + ipilimumab Ipilimumab	72 70	60 11	— 	8.9 months 4.7 months

5.3 Targeted Therapies

Two BRAFi are available for clinical use in the daily clinical practice, vemurafenib and dabrafenib.

Vemurafenib and dabrafenib are approved by the Food and Drug Administration (FDA) for the treatment of patients with unresectable or metastatic melanoma with a BRAF V600E mutation, as detected by an FDA-approved test.

The recommended dosages of vemurafenib and dabrafenib are 960 and 150 mg, respectively, both taken orally twice daily.

5.3.1 BRAFi in Monotherapy

- Vemurafenib versus dacarbazine (BRIM-3):
  - RR: 48% versus 5%
  - PFS: 5.6 versus 1.3 months
  - OS: 13.6 versus 9.7 months, without differences between V600E and V600K

- Dabrafenib versus dacarbazine (BREAK-3):
  - PFS: 5.1 versus 2.7 months.
  - RR: 50% versus 6%.
  - The significant clinical activity of dabrafenib was confirmed also in the phase 2 study BREAK-MB that included only patients with brain metastases showing a similar activity of the BRAFi when performed before or after a local treatment for brain metastases such as surgery or radiotherapy (28% vs. 20% response rate).
- Despite these advances in melanoma treatment, disease progression occurs in approximately 50% of patients within 6–7 months of commencing therapy with a BRAFi due to several mechanisms of resistance, most of which seem to rely on reactivation of the MAPK pathway.
- In order to avoid or delay resistance to a single drug, combination therapies with BRAFi and MEK inhibitors (MEKi) have been explored.

5.3.2 BRAFi + MEKi Combination Therapy

- Cobimetinib and trametinib are the two MEKi available for clinical use (Table 5.3.6).

TABLE 5.3.6   Results of the Main Randomized Trials Using Target Therapies (BRAF Inhibitors With/Out Anti-MEK)

Study	Design	Study arms	No. of patients	ORR (%)	PFS (median; months)	OS (median; months)
BRIM-3 [4]	Randomized	Dacarbazine	274	5	1.6	9.7
		Vemurafenib	275	48	5.3	13.6[a]
BREAK-3 [13]	Randomized	Dacarbazine	63	6	2.7	NR
		Dabrafenib	187	50	5.1	NR
Combi-D [5]	Randomized	Dabrafenib + trametinib	210	67	11	25.1
		Dabrafenib + placebo	210	51	8.8	18.7
Combi-V	Randomized	Dabrafenib + trametinib	352	64	11.4	Not reached
		Vemurafenib + placebo	352	51	7.3	17.2
Co-BRIM	Randomized	Vemurafenib + cobimetinib	247	68	9.9	Not reached
		Vemurafenib + placebo	248	45	6.2	Not reached

ORR, Overall response rate; OS, overall survival; PFS, progression-free survival.
[a]Data from McArthur GA, Chapman PB, Robert C, Larkin J, Haanen JB, Dummer R, Ribas A, Hogg D, Hamid O, Ascierto PA, Garbe C, Testori A, Maio M, Lorigan P, Lebbé C, Jouary T, Schadendorf D, O'Day SJ, Kirkwood JM, Eggermont AM, Dréno B, Sosman JA, Flaherty KT, Yin M, Caro I, Cheng S, Trunzer K, Hauschild A. Safety and efficacy of vemurafenib in BRAF(V600E) and BRAF(V600K) mutation-positive melanoma (BRIM-3): extended follow-up of a phase 3, randomised, open-label study. Lancet Oncol 2014;15(3):323–32. [14]

- Dabrafenib + trametinib versus dabrafenib only (Combi-D):
  - OS: 25.1 versus 18.7 months, respectively
  - PFS: 11 and 8.8 months, respectively
- Dabrafenib + trametinib versus vemurafenib only (Combi-V):
  - PFS: 11.4 versus 7.3 months
  - RR: 64% versus 51%
  - The hazard ratio for death in the combination therapy group: 0.69
- Vemurafenib + cobimetinib versus vemurafenib only:
  - PFS: 9.9 versus 6.2 months
  - RR: 68% versus 45%
  - Nine-month OS: 81% versus 73%

5.3.3 Adverse Events

- The mechanism of action of BRAFi not only is responsible for its clinical activity but is also the basis for the development of side effects and adverse events.
- Vemurafenib (Fig. 5.3.4): exanthema, photosensitivity, palmar-plantar dysesthesia or hand–foot syndrome (HFS), alopecia, pruritus, keratosis pilaris (KP)–like eruptions, actinic keratosis

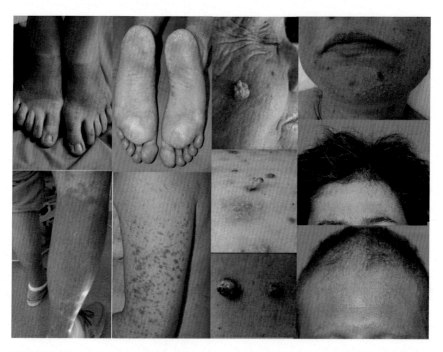

FIGURE 5.3.4 **Cutaneous side effects from anti-BRAF inhibitors.** From left to right and from the top to the bottom: photosensitivity reaction on the feet and lower limbs; plantar hyperkeratosis; erythematous papular eruption; seborrheic keratosis; verrucoid lesion; keratoacanthoma; milia on the face; hair modification and alopecia.

(AK), hyperkeratosis, skin papillomas, keratoacanthomas (KA), and cutaneous squamous cell carcinomas (SCC).
  - Photosensitivity is a specific side effect related to vemurafenib not related to the drug itself but to other compounds of the tablet.
- Dabrafenib: fever (frequently during the first weeks of treatment), hyperkeratosis, papilloma, alopecia, and palmar-plantar erythrodysesthesia syndrome.
- Trametinib: acneiform dermatitis or alopecia.
- Less is known about the cutaneous adverse events related to cobimetinib.
- The development of hyperkeratotic lesions and particularly AK, KA, and potentially SCC during BRAFi therapy is caused by activation of the MAPK pathway in keratinocytes with preexisting RAS mutations commonly found in chronically sun-damaged skin. Although BRAFi potently reduce RAF signaling in BRAF mutant cells, they cause increased CRAF signaling in wild-type cells, leading to the development of SCC.
- Thus the development of SCC is consequent to an abnormal and paradoxical activation of the MAP kinase pathway.
  - The concomitant administration of a MEKi reduces this activation and therefore has preventive effects on the development of SCC and KA.
  - When BRAF and MEKi drugs are combined, the development of cutaneous adverse events specific for each drug appears to be reduced.
  - Even if, generally, the combo regimens show fewer side effects with respect to the monotherapy with BRAFi, the association of dabrafenib and trametinib gives rise to a more frequent occurrence of fever.
- The two BRAFi available in the clinical practice are therefore characterized from one side by a substantially similar clinical activity profile, but on the other side by potentially relevant differences in the spectrum of adverse events, thus implying that the choice of one instead of the other should be done on the basis of the age and comorbidities of the patient to reduce the impact of toxicities.
- The side effects associated with target therapies and observed in the more relevant studies are summarized in Table 5.3.3 and compared with dose of immune checkpoint inhibitors.

5.4 c-Kit Inhibitors

Mutations and amplification of the KIT oncogene are more frequent in melanomas arising in the skin with chronic sun damage, acral sites, or mucosal melanomas.

- A series of laboratory evidence and preclinical studies demonstrated that hotspot mutations, most frequently constituted by substitutions at exons 11 and 13, induce a pathological activation of the KIT and thus an upregulation of the downstream signal transduction pathways, which are not only the MAP kinase but also the PI3K/AKT and JAK/STAT pathways.

- KIT gene expression has been correlated with activating mutations, which indicates the role of KIT in tumorigenesis in melanoma. Therefore, KIT has been suggested to be a potential therapeutic target for malignant melanoma.
- Several trials have been conducted using KIT-targeted tyrosine kinase inhibitors in melanoma in both selected and nonselected patient populations. Trials of imatinib demonstrated responses if KIT was mutated but not if it was wild-type and amplified. Other KIT inhibitors such as dasatinib, sunitinib, and nilotinib have also demonstrated responses in KIT-mutant melanomas (summarized in Table 5.3.7).
  - Taken together, however, these studies showed a percentage of responses around 20 and 30%, mostly of short duration without a significant impact on survival. Moreover, all these studies were performed on relatively small number of patients and no randomized trial is available.

It can be therefore hypothesized that durable responses in c-Kit mutant melanoma may require combination therapies selectively inhibiting downstream pathways (mainly the PI3K cascade which is the dominant effector of cell proliferation following c-Kit activation).

The limited clinical activity of targeting c-Kit implies that c-Kit mutant patients should be treated as first line with immune checkpoint inhibitors,

TABLE 5.3.7 Summary of Results of Studies Using c-Kit Inhibitors in Stage IV Metastatic Melanoma

	Guo (2011) [15]	Carvajal (2011) [16]	Hodi (2013) [17]	Lebbè (2014) [18]	Buchbinder (2015) [19]	Lee (2015) [20]
Patients	43	28	25	25	52	42
Drug	Imatinib	Imatinib	Imatinib	Nilotinib	Sunitinib	Nilotinib
RR (%)	23	16	29	20	7.7–9.7[a]	16.7
TTP	3.5 months	—	3.7 months	47.5% (6 months PFS)	—	34 weeks (median response duration)
Survival	54% (1-year OS)	11 months (median)	12.5 months (median)	67.2% (6 months OS)	6.4–8.6 months[a] (median)	—

OS, Overall survival; PFS, progression-free survival; RR, response rate; TTP, time to progression.
[a]Respectively, with or without KIT mutation.

and the potential of c-Kit inhibitors should be considered only after the failure of these regimens.

6 A COMPREHENSIVE SCENARIO FOR THE MANAGEMENT OF A PATIENT WITH STAGE IV METASTATIC MELANOMA AND FUTURE CHALLENGES

The introduction of new drugs, both immune checkpoint inhibitors and targeted therapies, has determined a complete change of paradigms and guidelines for the treatment of stage IV metastatic melanoma. Even if several guidelines have been proposed with potentially different indications, nevertheless a defined set of general principles can already be acknowledged (Fig. 5.3.5):

- Check for the mutation pattern in all patients with stage IV metastatic melanoma.
- Consider first the potential of surgery (limited disease extension with the possibility to completely resect the disease burden, prolonged disease-free survival, and a tumor volume doubling time potentially of >60 days).

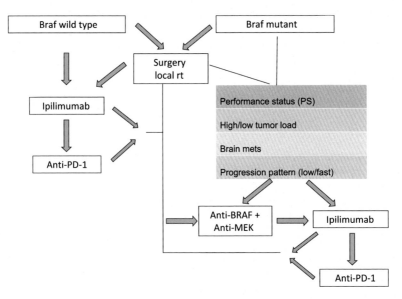

FIGURE 5.3.5 **A comprehensive scenario for the management of a patient with stage IV metastatic melanoma.**

- In BRAF wild-type patients, first-line treatment is represented by immune checkpoint inhibitors.
- In the presence of BRAF mutation, the choice of targeted therapies versus immunotherapy as first line should be based on the evaluation of patient characteristics and disease extension (performance status, high/low tumor load, brain mets, fast/low progression pattern).
- Always consider the possibility to add locally directed therapies (surgery, radiotherapy, electrochemotherapy) to improve the response rate (also considering the "abscopal" effect) or to treat a local progression.

A lot of open questions and challenges still exist, including the selection of patients more likely to benefit from immune therapy, the optimal sequencing of targeted and immune therapies, and the management of targeted therapies beyond progression. Future studies are clearly needed to clarify these issues.

Acknowledgment

The author thanks Prof. A.R. Filippi who contributed to this chapter.

References

[1] Hodi FS, O'Day SJ, McDermott DF, et al. Improved survival with ipilimumab in patients with metastatic melanoma. N Engl J Med 2010;363(8):711–23.

[2] Ribas A, Puzanov I, Dummer R, et al. Pembrolizumab versus investigator-choice chemotherapy for ipilimumab-refractory melanoma (KEYNOTE-002): a randomised, controlled, phase 2 trial. Lancet Oncol 2015;16(8):908–18.

[3] Hodi FS, Postow MA, Chesney JA, et al. Clinical response, progression-free survival (PFS), and safety in patients (pts) with advanced melanoma (MEL) receiving nivolumab (NIVO) combined with ipilimumab (IPI) vs IPI monotherapy in CheckMate 069 study. J Clin Oncol 2015;33(8):9004. ASCO Annual Meeting (May 29–June 2, 2015).

[4] Chapman PB, Hauschild A, Robert C, Haanen JB, Ascierto P, Larkin J, et al. BRIM-3 Study Group. Improved survival with vemurafenib in melanoma with BRAF V600E mutation. N Engl J Med 2011;364(26):2507–16.

[5] Long GV, Stroyakovskiy D, Gogas H, Levchenko E, de Braud F, Larkin J, et al. Dabrafenib and trametinib versus dabrafenib and placebo for Val600 BRAF-mutant melanoma: a multicentre, double-blind, phase 3 randomised controlled trial. Lancet 2015;386(9992):444–51.

[6] Larkin J, Ascierto PA, Dréno B, Atkinson V, Liszkay G, Maio M, et al. Combined vemurafenib and cobimetinib in BRAF-mutated melanoma. N Engl J Med 2014;371(20): 1867–76.

[7] Wolchok JD, Weber JS, Hamid O, et al. Ipilimumab efficacy and safety in patients with advanced melanoma: a retrospective analysis of HLA subtype from four trials. Cancer Immunol 2010;10:9.

[8] Robert C, Thomas L, Bondarenko I, et al. Ipilimumab plus dacarbazine for previously untreated metastatic melanoma. N Engl J Med 2011;364(26):2517–26.

[9] Schadendorf D, Hodi FS, Robert C, et al. Pooled analysis of long-term survival data from phase II and phase III trials of ipilimumab in unresectable or metastatic melanoma. J Clin Oncol 2015;33(17):1889–94.

[10] Robert C, Long GV, Brady B, et al. Nivolumab in previously untreated melanoma without BRAF mutation. N Engl J Med 2014;372(4):320–30.

[11] Robert C, Schachter J, Long GV, et al. Pembrolizumab versus Ipilimumab in advanced melanoma. N Engl J Med 2015;372:2521–32.

[12] Wolchok JD, Kluger H, Callahan MK, et al. Nivolumab plus ipilimumab in advanced melanoma. N Engl J Med 2013;369:122–33.

[13] Hauschild A, Grob JJ, Demidov LV, Jouary T, Gutzmer R, Millward M, et al. Dabrafenib in BRAF-mutated metastatic melanoma: a multicentre, open-label, phase 3 randomised controlled trial (BREAK-3). Lancet 2012;380(9839):358–65.

[14] McArthur GA, Chapman PB, Robert C, Larkin J, Haanen JB, Dummer R, et al. Safety and efficacy of vemurafenib in BRAF(V600E) and BRAF(V600K) mutation-positive melanoma (BRIM-3): extended follow-up of a phase 3, randomised, open-label study. Lancet Oncol 2014;15(3):323–32.

[15] Guo J, Si L, Kong Y, Flaherty KT, Xu X, Zhu Y, et al. Phase II, open-label, single-arm trial of imatinib mesylate in patients with metastatic melanoma harboring c-Kit mutation or amplification. J Clin Oncol 2011;29(21):2904–9.

[16] Carvajal RD, Antonescu CR, Wolchok JD, et al. KIT as a therapeutic target in metastatic melanoma. JAMA. 2011;305:2327–34.

[17] Hodi FS, Corless CL, Giobbie-Hurder A, et al. Imatinib for melanomas harboring mutationally activated or amplified KIT arising on mucosal, acral, and chronically sun-damaged skin. J Clin Oncol 2013;31:3182–90.

[18] Lebbe C, Chevret S, Jouary T, et al. Phase II multicentric uncontrolled national trial assessing the efficacy of nilotinib in the treatment of advanced melanomas with c-KIT mutation or amplification. J Clin Oncol 2014;32(Suppl. 15):9032.

[19] Buchbinder EI, Sosman JA, Lawrence DP, McDermott DF, Ramaiya NH, Van den Abbeele AD, et al. Phase 2 study of sunitinib in patients with metastatic mucosal or acral melanoma. Cancer 2015;121(22):4007–15.

[20] Lee SJ, Kim TM, Kim YJ, Jang KT, Lee HJ, Lee SN, et al. Phase II trial of nilotinib in patients with metastatic malignant melanoma harboring KIT gene aberration: a multi-center trial of Korean Cancer Study Group (UN10-06). Oncologist 2015;20(11):1312–9.

Follow-Up of Disease-Free Patients

Elvira Moscarella

University of Campania Luigi Vanvitelli, Naples, Italy; Arcispedale S. Maria
Nuova, IRCCS, Reggio Emilia, Italy

Follow-up of disease-free melanoma patients has two aims:

- Early detection of relapse through surveillance imaging
- Detection of eventual subsequent melanomas:
  - A previous history of having had a melanoma increases the risk of a second melanoma by approximately a factor of 10 and this risk is lifelong.

Cutaneous Melanoma. http://dx.doi.org/10.1016/B978-0-12-804000-3.00006-5

Current guidelines for follow-up include recommendations about frequency and modalities of both imaging exams and skin examinations but:

- Surveillance recommendations vary widely from country to country with respect to imaging studies and frequency of visits.
  - This is mainly due to the lack of evidence about the efficacy of follow-up programs (only monocentric, retrospective studies available).
- Therefore surveillance recommendations heavily depend on expert opinion.

Here we resume the most updated guidelines for follow-up with a focus on the efficacy of the proposed imaging exams, cost-effectiveness, and patients' perspective.

1 TIME TO RECURRENCE AND SURVIVAL

- Timing of relapse and survival rates vary according to stage.
- The majority of recurrences are recorded in the first 5 years of follow-up.
  - As a consequence, there is a general agreement for a higher intensity of follow-up visits during the first 5 years after melanoma diagnosis.
- Patients with early stage melanoma have extremely high DFS and DSS.
  - However, survival is not 100% and late recurrences may occur.
- Patients with stage III disease have more heterogeneous DFS and survival rates.
- Early detection of recurrence is associated with a higher survival rate.

2 COMPARISON OF CURRENT GUIDELINES

- Table 6.1 summarizes the follow-up guidelines developed in the European countries, the USA, and Australia.
  - Low-intensity strategies are preferably adopted in the United States, the United Kingdom, and Australia.
  - High-intensity strategies are adopted in Europe (except the United Kingdom).

In particular, the American Academy of Dermatology recommend imaging exams only based on symptoms. Guidelines for the Management of Melanoma in Australia and New Zealand (GMMANZ) emphasize the importance of self-examinations in patients properly trained to detect

TABLE 6.1   Comparison of Recommendation for Follow-Up of Melanoma Patients

Exams	National Comprehensive Cancer Network (NCCN)	National Collaborating Centre for Cancer (NCC-C)	German evidence-based guideline (malignant melanoma S3-guideline)	Guidelines for the Management of Melanoma in Australia and New Zealand (GMMANZ)
Clinical exam[a]	Lifelong for all stages at risk-adapted intervals *Stages Ia–IIa*: two times per year for the first 5 years, and then annually *Stages IIb–III*: three times per year for the first 2 years, then four times per year for 3 years, and then annually	*Stage Ia*: two to four times during the first year after completion of treatment, and then discharge *Stages Ib–III*: four times per year during the first 3 years, and then two times per year for 2 years	Lifelong for all stages at risk-adapted intervals *Stage Ia*: two times per year for the first 3 years, and then annually *Stages Ib–III*: four times per year for the first 3 years, then two times per year until 5 years, and then annually	Lifelong for all stages *Stage I*: two times per year during the first 5 years, and then annually *Stages II–III*: three to four times per year during the first 5 years, and then annually
Lymph node ultrasound	To be considered based on clinical exam *or* in patients not undergoing SLNB *or* in patients with positive SLNB and no completion lymphadenectomy	*Stage IIc* with no sentinel lymph node biopsy or *stage III* only if eligible for systemic therapy	*Stages Ib–III*	*Stages II–III* based on clinical exam
Abdominal ultrasound	Not recommended	*Stage IIc* with no sentinel lymph node biopsy or *stage III* only if eligible for systemic therapy	Based on symptoms	Not recommended
Chest X-ray	To be considered in *stages IIb–III* for 5 years	*Stage IIc* with no sentinel lymph node biopsy or *stage III* only if eligible for systemic therapy	Not recommended	Not recommended

(Continued)

TABLE 6.1   Comparison of Recommendation for Follow-Up of Melanoma Patients (*cont.*)

Exams	National Comprehensive Cancer Network (NCCN)	National Collaborating Centre for Cancer (NCC-C)	German evidence-based guideline (malignant melanoma S3-guideline)	Guidelines for the Management of Melanoma in Australia and New Zealand (GMMANZ)
CT scan *or* PET/CT	To be considered in *stages IIb–III* for 5 years	*Stage IIc* with no sentinel lymph node biopsy or *stage III* only if eligible for systemic therapy	*Stages IIc–III*	Not recommended
MRN	To be considered annually in *stages IIb–III* for 5 years for brain imaging	For brain imaging in young patients (<25 years) if brain metastasis is suspected	*Stages IIc–III* for detection of brain metastasis	Not recommended
S100B serum levels	Not recommended	Not recommended	*Stages Ib–III*	Not recommended

All guidelines consider follow-up recommendations for stage 0–III patients. For stage IV patients, individualized scheduled is suggested. NCCN guidelines were published in 2014. NCC-C guidelines were published in 2015. The German evidence-based guidelines (malignant melanoma S3-guideline) were published in 2013. The GMMANZ were published in 2008. The European Society of Medical Oncology (ESMO) and American Academy of Dermatology (AAD) guidelines are not reported in this table, because they do not follow a staging system, but provide general recommendations for monitoring patients at risk for recurrent and new disease. CT, Computed tomography; PET, positron emission tomography.

[a] *National Collaborative Center for Cancer (NCC-C) guidelines direct follow-up programs starting from stage Ia patients. Recommendation for stage 0 is to discharge patients following completion of treatment. No screening exam is offered to stage Ia–IIc patients with negative sentinel lymph node biopsy.*

recurrent disease. Ultrasound is among the recommended imaging techniques in patients with advanced disease, but only if performed by an experienced ultrasonographer. The National Comprehensive Cancer Network (NCCN) does not recommend routine imaging for stage IA–IIA disease. Five-year routine imaging is suggested to monitor patients with stage IIB–IV melanoma and includes chest X-ray, computed tomography (CT), and/or positron emission tomography (PET) scans every 3–12 months and annual magnetic resonance imaging (MRI) scans of the brain.

The European Society for Medical Oncology (ESMO) suggests performing CT and/or PET scan only in high-risk patients (i.e., those with thick primary tumors or following treatment of metastasis), for earlier detection of relapse. The German Cancer Society and the German Dermatologic Society suggest LN sonography and S100B dosage every 3–6 months for patients with stage IB–IV melanoma. Imaging studies, including CT, MRI, or PET scan, are suggested every 6 months in patients with stage IIC–IV melanoma. Abdominal sonography is suggested only in symptomatic patients.

- Table 6.2 displays the recommendations developed on the basis of the experience of a group of clinicians affiliated to referral centers dealing with melanoma diagnosis and management in Italy.
  - In all cases, the current guidelines suggest personalized follow-up for stage IV patients.

TABLE 6.2   Follow-Up Schedule by Stage

Exams	Stage 0	Stage Ia	Stage Ib	Stage II	Stage III
Clinical examination[a]	Once per year	6-Month interval for the first 5 years, and then annually	4-Month interval for the first 5 years, and then 6-month interval for 5 more years	4-Month interval for the first 5 years, and then 6-month interval for 5 more years	4-Month interval for the first 5 years, and then 6-month interval for 5 more years
Lymph node ultrasound	—	Every 12 months for 5 years or based on clinical exam	6- to 12-month interval for 5 years or based on clinical exam	12-Month interval for 5 years	Twice per year for 5 years, and then once per year for 5 more years (visits I and III in the year)
Abdominal ultrasound	—	—	—	Every 12 months for 5 years	Twice per year for 5 years, and then once per year for 5 more years (visits I and III in the year)
CT scan or PET/CT	—	—	—	Every 12 months for 5 years (at 6-month interval with ultrasound)	Once per year for 5 years (visit II in the year)

CT, Computed tomography; PET, positron emission tomography.
[a] *Clinical examination is intended to be lifelong independently from stage. Individual characteristics of the patient, such as total number of nevi, and personal and family history of melanoma, will influence the time interval. Clinical examination always includes dermoscopy.*

3 PATIENTS' PERSPECTIVE

- Patients' perspective is an important aspect to take into consideration when designing a follow-up protocol.
  - Patients highly value routine follow-up examinations.
  - Increased patients' anxiety related to follow-up exams has been reported, especially in cases of false-positive findings following imaging exams.
  - An adequate communication on the expectations of follow-up examinations is important.
  - Most melanoma guidelines recommend psychosocial intervention and education for all patients.

4 CLINICAL EXAM AND PATIENT EDUCATION

- Clinical evaluation is mandatory at any stage.
- Time frequencies of follow-up visits depend on the specific stage of disease.
- Clinical examination performed by a dermatologist should include:
  - A total-body skin evaluation for the identification of local recurrences, satellitosis, and in-transit or nodal metastases
  - The evaluation of patients' symptoms correlated to the disease progression
  - The clinical and dermoscopic examination of skin lesions, with the aim to identify eventual subsequent primary melanomas or other nonmelanoma skin cancer:
    - A recent multicenter study examined dermoscopy features of multiple primary melanomas (MPMs). MPM in a given patient had the same chance to look dermoscopically similar or different [1–3].
- Patients' education has to be part of the clinical exam, and is likely to play an important role in patient surveillance. It includes:
  - Information on how to perform regular self-exam (check the skin at least once a month, using good lighting, a full-length mirror, and a hand mirror)
  - Education on correct sun behavior

5 ULTRASOUND

- Ultrasound of regional lymph nodes has been demonstrated to have the highest accuracy and highest diagnostic validity to detect early regional relapse.

- Lymph node sonography is superior to palpation for the detection of lymph node metastases.
- Abdominal ultrasound can be added.
  - Its practicability with regard to quality, reproducibility, and cost depends on the examiner. Technical limitations result from the low depth of ultrasound wave penetration, as well as the possible shadows due to abdominal air and bones. Thus, especially intestinal and bone metastases cannot be detected early, and, in general, abdominal sonography has demonstrated a low sensitivity for the detection of small metastases.

6 CT SCAN AND PET/CT

- CT allows detecting distant recurrence in 18.5% of stage II and 33% of stage III disease.
  - However, the effectiveness of CT scan was limited by the high number of false-positive rates (20%), resulting in an overall low positive predictive value.
- Total-body CT scan should be considered in the follow-up of patients with higher risk of developing distant metastasis.

7 CHEST X-RAY AND BLOOD TESTS

- Conventional chest X-ray has been proven to be clearly inferior to CT for the detection of pulmonary metastases.
- Similarly, for blood tests, such as S100 protein and LDH values, low positive predictive values have been demonstrated.

8 FAMILY HISTORY OF MELANOMA AND CDKN2A MUTATION

- Patients with family history of melanoma and/or MPMs, in which CDKN2A mutation is present, carry higher risk of developing both additional primaries and pancreatic cancer.
- For these patients, abdominal sonography and blood level of C19.9 cancer marker performed every 6 months were proposed in addition to the clinical and imaging examinations at any stage in the recently developed Italian recommendations.
  - However, no international consensus exists on this surveillance approach, and some authors recommend MRI to detect early stage pancreatic cancer.

9 COST-EFFECTIVENESS

- Evaluation of cost-effectiveness is particularly difficult, considering such extreme variations in clinical practice.
- A recent prospective study was conducted in Germany, following a large and representative cohort of melanoma patients for 4 years since the initial melanoma diagnosis. The value of the follow-up care was critically appraised by calculating the costs of the follow-up for patients without tumor recurrence. The study concluded that for low-risk melanoma patients with stage I–IIB melanoma and in situ melanoma patients, follow-up frequency and investigations can be reduced in Germany and thus expenses saved.

10 CONCLUSIONS

- Currently, no universally adopted schedules exist for monitoring patients with cutaneous melanoma.
- Studies evaluating the economic burden of the surveillance program should be conducted in order to validate the current approaches.
- Finally, patients' perspective should be taken into higher consideration. Increased patients' anxiety related to follow-up exams has been reported, especially in cases of false-positive findings following imaging exams.

References

[1] Network NCC. NCCN clinical practice guidelines in oncology: melanoma, <http://www.nccn.org/professionals/physician_gls/pdf/melanoma.pdf>.

[2] Party ACNMGRW. Clinical practice guidelines for the management of melanoma in Australia and New Zealand, <http://www.nhmrc.gov.au/_files_nhmrc/file/publications/synopses/cp111.pdf>.

[3] Pflugfelder A, Kochs C, Blum A, et al. Malignant melanoma S3-guideline "diagnosis, therapy and follow-up of melanoma". J Dtsch Dermatol Ges 2013;11(Suppl. 6):1–116.

Further Reading

Altekruse SF, Kosary CL, Krapcho M, editors. SEER cancer statistics review, 1975–2007. Bethesda, MD: National Cancer Institute; 2010http://seer.cancer.gov/csr/1975_2007.

American Cancer Society. Cancer facts & figures 2013. Atlanta: American Cancer Society; 2013.

Argenziano G, Soyer HP, Chimenti S, et al. Dermoscopy of pigmented skin lesions: results of a consensus meeting via the internet. J Am Acad Dermatol 2003;48(5):679–93.

Bafounta ML, Beauchet A, Chagnon S, Saiag P. Ultrasonography or palpation for detection of melanoma nodal invasion: a meta-analysis. Lancet Oncol 2004;5:673–80.

Bichakjian CK, Halpern AC, Johnson TM, et al. Guidelines of care for the management of primary cutaneous melanoma. American Academy of Dermatology. J Am Acad Dermatol 2011;65:1032–47.

Bowles TL, Xing Y, Hu CY, Mungovan KS, et al. Conditional survival estimates improve over 5 years for melanoma survivors with node-positive disease. Ann Surg Oncol 2010;17:2015–23.

Brown RE, Stromberg AJ, Hagendoorn LJ, et al. Surveillance after surgical treatment of melanoma: futility of routine chest radiography. Surgery 2010;148:711–6.

Dummer R, Hauschild A, Guggenheim M, et al. Melanoma: ESMO clinical practice guidelines of care for the diagnosis, treatment, and follow-up. Ann Oncol 2010;21(Suppl. 5):194–7.

Dummer R, Panizzon R, Bloch PH, Burg G. Updated Swiss guidelines for the treatment and follow-up of cutaneous melanoma. Dermatology 2005;210:39–44.

Fong ZV, Tanabe KK. Comparison of melanoma guidelines in the U.S.A., Canada, Europe, Australia and New Zealand: a critical appraisal and comprehensive review. Br J Dermatol 2014;170:20–30.

Francken A, Bastiaannet E, Hoekstra H. Follow-up in patients with localised primary cutaneous melanoma. Lancet Oncol 2005;6:608–21.

Francken AB, Accortt NA, Shaw HM, et al. Follow-up schedules after treatment for malignant melanoma. Br J Surg 2008;95:1401–7.

Garbe C. Prospective evaluation of a follow-up schedule in cutaneous melanoma patients: recommendations for an effective follow-up strategy. J Clin Oncol 2003;21:520–9.

Goggins WB, Tsao H. A population-based analysis of risk factors for a second primary cutaneous melanoma among melanoma survivors. Cancer 2003;97:639–43.

Hengge UR, Wallerand A, Stutzki A, Kockel N. Cost-effectiveness of reduced follow-up in malignant melanoma. J Dtsch Dermatol Ges 2007;5:898–907.

Hofmann U, Szedlak M, Rittgen W, Jung EG, Schadendorf D. Primary staging and follow-up in melanoma patients—monocenter evaluation of methods, costs and patient survival. Br J Cancer 2002;87:151–7.

Holterhues C, van de Poll-Franse LV, de Vries E, Neumann HA, Nijsten TE. Melanoma patients receive more follow-up care than current guideline recommendations: a study of 546 patients from the general Dutch population. J Eur Acad Dermatol Venereol 2012;26:1389–95.

Kalimullah FA, Brown CW. Compliance with follow-up among patients with melanoma and non-melanoma skin cancers. Dermatol Online J 2014;20.

Kang S, Barnhill RL, Mihm MC Jr, Sober AJ. Multiple primary cutaneous melanomas. Cancer 1992;70:1911–6.

Leiter U, Buettner PG, Eigentler TK, et al. Hazard rates for recurrent and secondary cutaneous melanoma: an analysis of 33,384 patients in the German Central Malignant Melanoma Registry. J Am Acad Dermatol 2012;66:37–45.

Leiter U, Marghoob AA, Lasithiotakis K, et al. Costs of the detection of metastases and follow-up examinations in cutaneous melanoma. Melanoma Res 2009;19:50–7.

Livingstone E, Krajewski C, Eigentler TK, et al. Prospective evaluation of follow-up in melanoma patients in Germany—results of a multicentre and longitudinal study. Eur J Cancer 2015;51(5):653–67.

Lynch HT, Fusaro RM, Lynch JF, Brand R. Pancreatic cancer and the FAMMM syndrome. Fam Cancer 2008;7(1):103–12.

Marzuka-Alcalá A, Gabree MJ, Tsao H. Melanoma susceptibility genes and risk assessment. Methods Mol Biol 2014;1102:381–93.

McKenna DB, Marioni JC, Lee RJ, et al. A comparison of dermatologists', surgeons' and general practitioners' surgical management of cutaneous melanoma. Br J Dermatol 2004;151(3):636–44.

National Collaborating Centre for Cancer (UK). Melanoma: assessment and management. London: National Institute for Health and Care Excellence (UK); 2015.

Meyers MO, Yeh JJ, Frank J, et al. Method of detection of initial recurrence of stage II/III cutaneous melanoma: analysis of the utility of follow-up staging. Ann Surg Oncol 2009;16:941–7.

Mocellin S, Zavagno G, Nitti D. The prognostic value of serum S100B in patients with cutaneous melanoma: a meta-analysis. Int J Cancer 2008;123(10):2370–6.

Mooney MM. Impact on survival by method of recurrence detection in stage I and II cutaneous melanoma. Ann Surg Oncol 1998;5(1):54–63.

Moscarella E, Rabinovitz H, Puig S, et al. Multiple primary melanomas: do they look the same? Br J Dermatol 2013;168(6):1267–72.

Poo-Hwu WJ, Ariyan S, Lamb L, et al. Follow-up recommendations for patients with American Joint Committee on Cancer stages I–III malignant melanoma. Cancer 1999;86:2252–8.

Romano E, Scordo M, Dusza SW, Coit DG, Chapman PB. Site and timing of first relapse in stage III melanoma patients: implications for follow-up guidelines. J Clin Oncol 2010;28(18):3042–7.

Rueth NM, Xing Y, Chiang YJ, et al. Is surveillance imaging effective for detecting surgically treatable recurrences in patients with melanoma? A comparative analysis of stage-specific surveillance strategies. Ann Surg 2014;259(6):1215–22.

Rychetnik L, McCaffery K, Morton R, Irwig L. Psychosocial aspects of post-treatment follow-up for stage I/II melanoma: a systematic review of the literature. Psychooncology 2013;22(4):721–36.

Themstrup L, Jemec GE, Lock-Andersen J. Patients highly value routine follow-up of skin cancer and cutaneous melanoma. Dan Med J 2013;60(10):A4713.

Tsao H, Cosimi AB, Sober AJ. Ultra-late recurrence (15 years or longer) of cutaneous melanoma. Cancer 1997;79:2361–70.

Turner RM, Bell KJ, Morton RL, et al. Optimizing the frequency of follow-up visits for patients treated for localized primary cutaneous melanoma. J Clin Oncol 2011;29:4641–6.

Uren RF, Howman-Giles R, Thompson JF, et al. High-resolution ultrasound to diagnose melanoma metastases in patients with clinically palpable lymph nodes. Australas Radiol 1999;43:148–52.

Vasen HF, Wasser M, van Mil A, et al. Magnetic resonance imaging surveillance detects early-stage pancreatic cancer in carriers of a p16-Leiden mutation. Gastroenterology 2011;140(3):850–6.

Xing Y, Bronstein Y, Ross MI, et al. Contemporary diagnostic imaging modalities for the staging and surveillance of melanoma patients: a meta-analysis. J Natl Cancer Inst 2011;103:129–42.

Yancovitz M, Finelt N, Warycha MA, et al. Role of radiologic imaging at the time of initial diagnosis of stage T1b–T3b melanoma. Cancer 2007;110:1107–14.

Zalaudek I, Docimo G, Argenziano G. Using dermoscopic criteria and patient-related factors for the management of pigmented melanocytic nevi. Arch Dermatol 2009;145(7):816–26.

Zimmer L, Haydu LE, Menzies AM, et al. Incidence of new primary melanomas after diagnosis of stage III and IV melanoma. J Clin Oncol 2014;32:816–23.

CHAPTER

7

Special Clinical Situations

7.1

The Histopathological Gray Zone

Gerardo Ferrara

Macerata General Hospital, Macerata, Italy

1 INTRODUCTION

Professional histological examination of hematoxylin and eosin (H&E)–stained tissue sections from routinely processed skin biopsy samples is still the undisputable mainstay for the diagnosis of melanocytic skin neoplasms. One major problem, however, is that the histopathological diagnosis of melanoma is not based on the search of a single (or a few), objective, and easily reproducible morphological diagnostic feature(s) but rather, it is born by a constellation of diagnostic criteria whose implementation, meaning, and relative weight considerably vary case by case and is responsible for a worrisome list of diagnostic pitfalls (Table 7.1.1). Thus, the histopathological diagnosis of melanocytic skin neoplasms, being based on the simultaneous evaluation of several criteria, is no more than an *assessment of probability* and, as such, is often matter of a sizable disagreement and interobserver variability [1]. In addition, and even more importantly, the time-honored "unifying concept of melanoma" (melanoma as a single entity evolving with a well-defined and repetitive "sequence of events") [2] has been questioned, because both clinicopathological [3] and molecular studies [4] point toward the existence of low-grade melanocytic malignancies different from "conventional" melanoma.

For all the previous discussion, in recent years the traditional "dichotomic" (white vs. black; benign vs. malignant) approach to the diagnosis of melanocytic skin neoplasms is increasingly becoming less popular [5]: All melanocytic tumors might be best distributed along a spectrum, with a "gray zone" being in between the "white" (completely benign) and the "black" (overtly malignant) ends [6]. From a practical point of view, we can typify the "gray zone" as composed of

TABLE 7.1.1   Main Settings of Diagnostic Difficulties in Melanocytic Skin Neoplasms

1. Unrecognized melanoma on partial (shave/punch) biopsies
2. Nevoid melanoma versus "common" or "congenital" compound/dermal nevus
3. Desmoplastic melanoma versus desmoplastic nevus versus scar
4. Recurrent/persistent nevus versus (recurrent) melanoma
5. Spindle cell melanoma versus spindle cell nevus
6. (Spitzoid) melanoma versus Spitz nevus
7. Superficial spreading melanoma versus "dysplastic" nevus
8. Superficial spreading melanoma versus haloed nevus
9. Melanoma (in special site) versus nevus with site-related atypia
10. Superficial spreading melanoma versus compound nevus with regression-like fibrosis
11. Melanoma with regression versus melanosis
12. Melanoma in situ in chronic sun-damaged skin versus melanocytic hyperplasia
13. Dermal melanoma over congenital nevus versus proliferative nodule in congenital nevus
14. Cellular blue nevus versus dendritic cell (animal-type) melanoma versus blue nevus-like metastatic melanoma

the following: (1) melanocytic neoplasms with conflicting histopathological criteria (intermediate morphology); (2) melanocytic neoplasms with unpredictable biological behavior (intermediate biology). It must be preliminarily underlined that the former category is much broader than the latter and that an "intermediate biology" is invariably associated with an "intermediate morphology," with the reverse being not necessarily true [1].

2 MELANOCYTIC NEOPLASMS WITH CONFLICTING HISTOPATHOLOGICAL CRITERIA

The existence of "morphologically intermediate" but biologically benign melanocytic neoplasms is implicit to the assumption that, along with some deceptively bland melanomas (see Chapter 3.4), there are several nevi that, to various extents, can be "atypical," that is, deviating from a stereotypical (normal) counterpart [7]. These nevi are listed in Table 7.1.2.

2.1 Common (Compound/Dermal) Nevi

- Defined as "mitotically active," when at least one mitotic figure is found within their dermal component. Such an occurrence has been surprisingly documented in up to 42.8% of cases with the aid of immunohistochemistry [8].
  - In most cases, the mitotic figures are single and located within the superficial portion of the dermis. More than two mitotic figures per

TABLE 7.1.2   List of Possibly "Atypical" Nevi

1. Common nevi
2. "Dysplastic" nevi
3. Recurrent nevi:
   a. Following incomplete excision ("Ackerman's pseudomelanomas")
   b. Following chronic trauma ("sclerosing nevi with pseudomelanomatous features")
4. Congenital nevi biopsied shortly after birth:
   a. With pagetoid spread
   b. With lentiginous growth
   c. With proliferative nodule(s)
5. Spitz and Reed nevi
6. BAP1 mutation-associated melanocytic nevi:
   a. Syndromic
   b. Sporadic
7. Common/cellular blue nevi
8. Nevi with associated/superimposed dermatosis:
   a. Nevi with eczematous changes (Meyerson's)
   b. Nevi associated with lichen sclerosus
   c. Nevi associated with vacuolar interface dermatitis
   d. Nevi associated with psoriasis
   e. Nevi associated with mycosis fungoides
9. Nevi in special sites (nevi with site-related atypia):
   a. Genital area
   b. Acral skin
   c. Scalp
   d. Ankle
   e. Flexural areas (axilla, groin, knee, umbilicus, pubis, scrotum, perineum, elbow)
   f. Breast/milk line
   g. Ear
   h. Conjunctiva

lesion can be usually explained by young patient age, pregnancy, traumatization, or inflammation [8].

   – Mitotic activity is not enough to switch the histopathological diagnosis into melanoma; nevertheless we use mitotic figures, even at the junction, as a tiebreaker criterion in conflicting morphological settings.

- Compound/dermal nevi with congenital-like can frequently display "angiotropism" (subendothelial herniation or intralymphatic misplacement of melanocytes), a feature which does not imply malignancy [9]. Instead, we are personally very careful when we see a similar finding in the context of a spitzoid melanocytic tumor [10].
- Intradermal or largely intradermal melanocytic nevi of the type often found on the skin of the face (so-called Miescher's nevi) exceptionally demonstrate dermal melanocytes with large, irregularly shaped smudgy hyperchromatic nuclei similar to those seen in ancient

neurofibromas and schwannomas; thrombosis, fibrin deposition, interstitial mucin, "patchy" (perivascular) lymphocytic infiltration, and fibrosis are often associated [11].

2.2 Dysplastic Nevi

- These were initially described as putative precursors of melanoma, first in melanoma-prone families [12] and then even in single patients with no personal/familial history of melanoma [13].
- The criteria adopted to define a nevus as "dysplastic" are far from being homogeneous and reproducible. According to the WHO 2006 [14] definition, the major histopathological criteria include architectural and cytological features:
  - Size ≥4 mm
  - Junctional component often adjacent to a compound nevomelanocytic component (the so-called "shoulder effect" or "shouldering")
  - Confluent nests ("bridging") and/or single ("lentiginous") melanocytes mainly near the tips but also at the sides of elongated rete ridges
  - Stromal reactions (concentric and lamellar fibroplasia; newly formed vessels; patchy perivascular lymphocytic infiltrate; melanophages)
  - Cytologic atypia, graded as mild or moderate:
    - Roundish and nonhyperchromatic nuclei characterize both mild and moderate dysplasia, with the latter also disclosing nuclei characterized by a size exceeding the size of the nuclei of keratinocytes and/or by small nucleoli. The cytoplasms of melanocytes are usually scanty in mild dysplasia and only focally abundant, with dusty pigmentation, in moderate dysplasia.
- The increasing quantitative representation of these morphological criteria places such tumors into a "spectrum" of increasing degree of histopathological atypia (Fig. 7.1.1).
  - The right end of this spectrum ("nevi with severe dysplasia," typified by melanocytes with hyperchromatic and irregular/angulated nuclei, prominent nucleoli, and/or abundant and dusty pigmented cytoplasms throughout the entire lesion) merges with (superficial spreading) melanoma.
  - This means that only a minority of "dysplastic nevi" are histopathologically atypical enough to show truly conflicting diagnostic criteria [1].
  - Moreover, and even more important, the assumption that the increasing degree of dysplasia is related to an increasing risk of evolution into melanoma is undemonstrated to date, also because most melanomas arise de novo, rather than in association with a nevus [15].

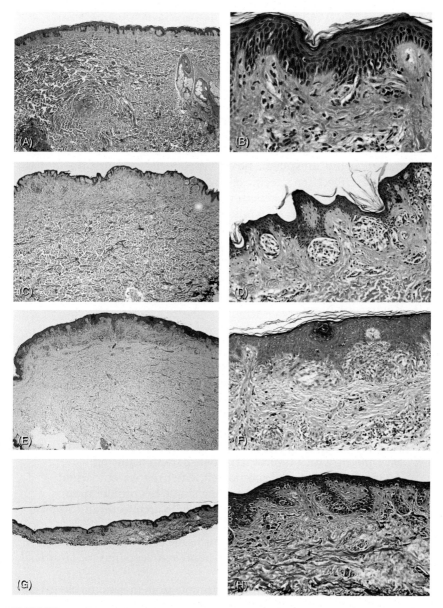

FIGURE 7.1.1 **Grading of dysplastic nevi.** (A and B) A "junctional nevus with mild dysplasia" with fibroplasia around the contours of the rete ridges (concentric fibroplasia), and junctional nests made by melanocytes whose nuclei are smaller than the nuclei of keratinocytes. (C and D) A "compound nevus with moderate dysplasia" characterized by concentric fibroplasia and junctional melanocytes whose nuclei are larger than the nuclei of keratinocytes. (E and F) A "compound nevus with moderate dysplasia" characterized by a multilayered ("lamellar") dermal fibroplasia. (G and H) A shave biopsy from a "junctional nevus with severe dysplasia"; the growth pattern is prevailingly lentiginous and melanocytes show irregular/angulated hyperchromatic nuclei.

TABLE 7.1.3   The WHO 2006 Criteria for the Diagnosis of "Dysplastic Nevus Syndrome"

- At least 100 nevi
- At least three clinically atypical nevi
- At least two nevi on the scalp
- One nevus on the buttock or at least three nevi on the dorsa of the feet
- At least two iris nevi

The diagnosis is made if at least three criteria are met.

- In our view, the "dysplastic nevus" diagnostic category, if adopted, must be ascribed to a specific entity as identified by a reference standard (e.g., the WHO 2006 criteria [14]); it must not be used for purposes of defensive medicine alone; it must not be used as a criterion to assess the risk of a given patient to develop a melanoma.
- Parenthetically, the "dysplastic nevus syndrome" is diagnosed on the basis of clinical criteria and not on the basis of the histopathological diagnosis of "dysplastic nevus" (Table 7.1.3).

2.3 Recurrent Nevi

- These are characterized by atypical clinicopathological features [16], as already discussed in Chapter 3.4.
- "Chronically recurrent nevi" following chronic unnoticed trauma have been described mainly in the convex area of the back of young to middle-aged patients: these neoplasms have been termed "sclerosing nevi with pseudomelanomatous features," "nevi with regression-like fibrosis," and "dysplastic nevi with florid fibroplasia" [17–21].
  - Histopathologically, these neoplasms are usually large and asymmetric with a typical "trizonal" pattern featuring
  - An irregular junctional component with irregular epidermal hyperplasia and areas of prevailing single cell proliferation
  - A significant area of dermal sclerosis with architecturally atypical melanocytic nests
  - A residual, bland-appearing nevus tissue (very often with congenital nevus-like features) around and deep into the cicatricial tissue (Fig. 7.1.2)
  - The differential features of these tumors from melanoma are given in Table 7.1.4. In addition to the histopathological criteria, we underline the importance of the clinicopathological correlation: in our experience, these benign tumors are often present as multiple lesions in the same patient ("signature nevi" [22]), and this is a clue of benignity.

Atypical features in congenital nevi biopsied shortly after birth have been already illustrated in Chapter 3.4.

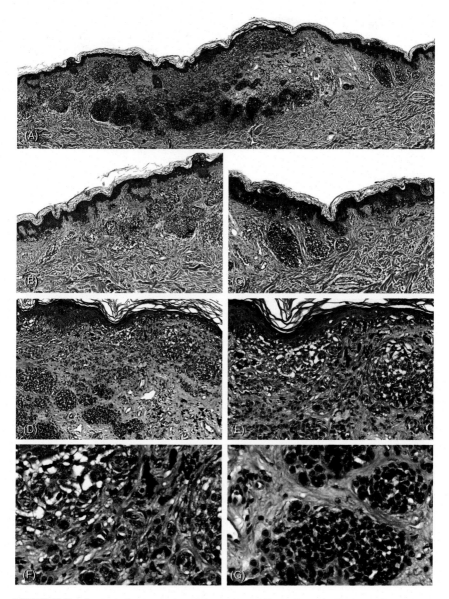

FIGURE 7.1.2 **A melanocytic neoplasm removed from the scapular area of a 33-year-old woman.** (A) The lesion is asymmetric because of the presence of a wide area of regression-like fibrosis. (B and C) In spite of the overall asymmetry, the lateral edges of the proliferation are remarkably similar. (D and E) Within the fibrotic area, there is flattening of the dermoepidermal junction with wide and irregular confluence of junctional nests of melanocytes. (F and G) While the superficial portion of the lesion shows some features of cytologic atypia, the deep dermal component is very bland, with a congenital nevus-like pattern. Histopathological diagnosis: sclerosing nevus with pseudomelanomatous features (compound nevus with egression-like fibrosis).

TABLE 7.1.4 Differential Features of Sclerosing Nevus With Pseudomelanomatous Features From Cutaneous Melanoma

	SNPMF	RPM	RM
Asymmetry	+	++	++
Poor lateral circumscription	−/+	++	++
Prevailing single cell junctional proliferation	+/++	++	++
Irregular architecture of nests	+	++	++
Pagetoid spreading	−/+	++	++
Epidermal atrophy/consumption	−/+	+/++	+/++
Maturation	++	−	−
Cytologic atypia	−/+	+/++	+/++
Deep dermal mitoses	−	+/++	+/++
Fibrosis	++ (tidy, in parallel bundles)	++ (more or less cellular)	++ (pale, irregular, with "wiry" bundles)
Melanophages	−/+	+/++	+/++
Lymphocytic infiltrate	−/+ (patchy)	+/++ (patchy or lichenoid)	+/++ (lichenoid)
Vertically oriented vessels	+/++	−/+	++
Fibrosis/inflammation beyond the lateral borders of the lesion	−	++	+/++
Elastic fibers	Candelabra-like within the papillary dermis	Compressed at the base of the tumor	Compressed at the base of the tumor

+, Usually mild; −, usually absent; ++, usually moderate to marked; RM, regressing primary melanoma; RPM, recurrent/persistent melanoma; SNPMF, sclerosing nevus with pseudomelanomatous features (nevus with regression-like fibrosis, dysplastic nevus with florid fibroplasia).

2.4 Spitz Nevi

- "Typically atypical"
- When junctional/thin compound are characterized by the following:
  - Plaque shape.
  - Well-circumscribed intraepidermal proliferation mostly composed of sharply demarcated melanocytic nests within a more or less hyperplastic epidermis.
  - Large spindle and/or epithelioid melanocytes arranged perpendicular and parallel to the skin surface; they are highly

cohesive and not destroy the nearby keratinocytes; therefore, a semilunar cleavage is often evident around nests ("capping") and even around the few single intraepidermal melanocytes ("microcapping") [23].

- Transepidermal elimination of nests is common and can be responsible for the complete involution of these lesions [24].
- Melanin pigment is present mainly within spindle cells, dermal melanophages (often arranged in a band-like fashion), and single intraepidermal dendritic melanocytes.

• When a sizable dermal component is present:
  - Dome shape.
  - Regularly spaced dermal nests and cords of cells.
  - A fascicular pattern of growth can be found and has been consistently associated with ALK immunopositivity and ALK (2p23) gene rearrangement (with the fusion partner being TPM3 on 1q21 or DCTN1 on 2p13) [25].
  - Maturation is at least focally seen.
  - Mitoses may be found, but virtually never in large number and never close to the base of the lesion.

• Some histological variants of Spitz nevus are on record (Table 7.1.5): awareness of these variants is important in order to avoid overdiagnosis of melanoma.

• We have proposed a four-tiered "grading system" for spitzoid neoplasms: in between Spitz nevus and spitzoid melanoma is a "gray zone" encompassing atypical Spitz nevus and (atypical) Spitz tumor, with the former being characterized by a slight architectural disarrangement within the superficial component of the tumor (slight asymmetry; lack of sharp lateral circumscription of the

TABLE 7.1.5   Histological Variants of Spitz Nevus

- Pigmented spindle cell (Reed nevus)
- Early
- Pagetoid
- Desmoplastic/sclerotic/hyalinizing
- Fascicular
- Halo
- Plaque-type (of the lower limbs)
- Epithelioid cell nevus of the thighs (of women)
- Polypoid
- Pseudoepitheliomatous/verrucous
- Angiomatous
- Pseudogranulomatous
- Plexiform
- Tubular
- Myxoid
- Combined

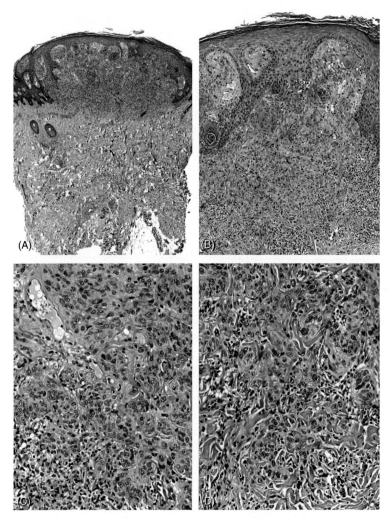

FIGURE 7.1.3 **A compound spitzoid tumor removed from the buttock of a 24-year-old woman.** (A) The lesion is small, symmetric, and dome-shaped. (B) There is an irregular confluence of the nests of melanocytes within the superficial dermis. (C and D) The proliferation shows a reduction in the size of the nests and the size of the cells toward the depth. Dermal mitotic figures are not found. Histopathological diagnosis: atypical Spitz nevus.

junctional component; focal epidermal thinning; slight confluence of the superficial nests) (Fig. 7.1.3) [23,26].

- By definition, both Spitz nevus and atypical Spitz nevus lack ulceration, large dermal sheets of cells, and relevant mitotic activity, which are features of a "tumorigenic" neoplasm (see the subsequent text).
- A narrow reexcision can be proposed for atypical Spitz nevi [23,26].

2.5 BAP1 Mutation-Associated Melanocytic Nevi (BAP1-Inactivated Nevi, BAPomas, Wiesner Nevi)

- These were first described as multiple fibroma-like amelanotic skin tumors in carriers of germline inactivating mutation of the BAP1 gene on 3p21 [27].
- Such a germline mutation was also identified as predisposing to uveal and cutaneous melanoma as well as to internal malignancies (mesothelioma, clear cell renal cell carcinoma, lung adenocarcinoma, head–neck squamous cell carcinoma, breast carcinoma, myelodysplasia, medulloblastoma, meningioma, head–neck squamous cell carcinoma) [28].
  - Shortly after, even sporadic melanocytic tumors of the skin were found to harbor biallelic inactivating mutations of the BAP1 gene [29].
- The histopathological picture of these melanocytic proliferations is a dermal-based nodular/polypoid growth of moderately pleomorphic epithelioid cells with centrally or eccentrically placed oval to kidney bean–shaped nuclei and abundant glassy eosinophilic, often inclusion-like cytoplasms.
  - BAP1 mutation-associated melanocytic proliferations span over a morphobiological spectrum ranging from mildly atypical proliferations to morphologically clear-cut melanomas.
- The less atypical tumors are characterized by the following:
  - Loosely arranged dermal nests separated by small amounts of stroma and interspersed lymphocytes
  - Mitotic figures usually not found (Fig. 7.1.4)
  - Often "combined," with evidence of a good "merging" with a bland-appearing nevomelanocytic component (in such a "combined" setting, the lymphocytic infiltrate is typically confined to the epithelioid cell component)
  - Lacking of "tumorigenic" features (ulceration, large dermal sheets of cells, and relevant mitotic activity) [30]
  - Immunohistochemical evidence of loss of the constitutive nuclear staining for the BAP1 protein [30]
  - BRAFV600E mutation in about 70% of cases, which can be also detected as a positive cytoplasmic immunostain with the VE1 antibody [31]:
    - This feature is seldom found in Spitz nevi and tumors, thereby confirming that BAP1 mutation-associated melanocytic proliferations, albeit showing a somewhat "spitzoid" cytomorphology, must be probably set apart from Spitz nevi and tumors [32]. Nevertheless, we think that the management of these tumors should cautiously follow the same rules as for spitzoid neoplasms.

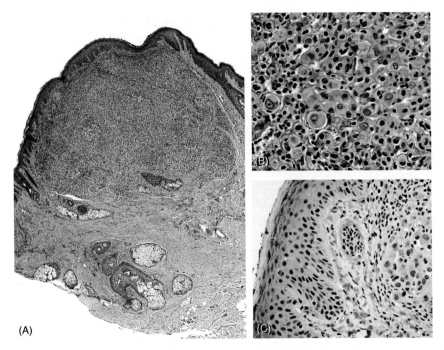

(A)   (B)   (C)

FIGURE 7.1.4 **A nodular lesion of the nasolabial fold in a 48-year-old woman.**
(A) The tumor is dermal-based, multinodular, nodular, with scattered inflammatory cells.
(B) The cytomorphological detail, featuring monotonously atypical epithelioid cells, often with eccentric nuclei and inclusion-like cytoplasms. (C) Constitutive nuclear expression of the BAP1 protein is lost within the dermal tumor. Histopathological diagnosis: BAPoma, benign.

2.6 Atypical (Cellular) Blue Nevi

- The histopathological pattern of common blue nevus is defined as "dendritic–sclerotic": this is typified by the presence of elongated, finely branched, heavily pigmented dendritic melanocytes interspersed with some melanophages among thickened bundles of collagen in the mid and the upper dermis with a readily appreciable "grenz zone"; not uncommonly, blue nevus is mainly composed of oval, often plump, melanocytes almost devoid of any pigment (hypoamelanotic blue nevus) [33–35].
- On the other hand, the histological pattern of "cellular" blue nevus is characterized by dendritic melanocytes together with "pale" islands of nonpigmented epithelioid (type A), nevocytic (type B), or spindle (type C) cells; the tumor often bulges into the subcutaneous fat as a nodular downgrowth with a typical clapper-like silhouette [35].

- In our view, given the definitions as specified previously, an atypical (cellular) blue nevus is basically a "mitotically active" (1–2 mitoses/mmq) blue nevus; in addition, we consider as "atypical" a cellular blue nevus with areas of predominant infiltration of melanophages and/or with "pale" islands composed of cells with prominent nucleoli. Nontraumatic ulceration, necrosis, and mitotic rate >2 mmq^{-1} are instead features of malignancy ("malignant blue nevus" or "blue nevus-like melanoma") [35].
- If defined according to these strict criteria, the prognosis of atypical (cellular) blue nevus is invariably good [34]: as with atypical Spitz nevus, a narrow reexcision has to be considered.

2.7 Nevi With Associated/Superimposed Dermatosis

- They show various degrees of architectural disturbance not due to the melanocytic proliferation itself.
- The best known phenomenon is the eosinophilic spongiotic (eczematous) reaction or Meyerson's phenomenon; although initially described in nevi [36] and by far more common under benign conditions, it can be found even in melanoma [37].
- In Meyerson's nevi, however, cytologic atypia, if present, is never marked or widespread and the upward spread of melanocytes is mainly central and within the foci of spongiosis [38].
- Even nevi from patients with psoriasis can show a relevant upward spread of melanocytes, probably as a result of the speeding of the epidermal transit time of the patients.
- Melanocytic nevi associated with lichen sclerosus are mainly, although not exclusively, found in the genital area. They are characterized by confluent nests varying in size and shape, horizontal "clefting" at the junction, and upward spread of nested and single melanocytes; in addition, the dermal changes (fibrosis, lichenoid lymphocytic infiltrate, and pigment incontinence with melanophages) may suggest regression of melanoma. The clinical picture as well as the presence of changes of lichen sclerosus well beyond the melanocytic proliferation is a good clue to the diagnosis [39].

2.8 Nevi in Special Sites (Nevi With Site-Related Atypia)

- Benign melanocytic proliferations whose atypical architectural and cytological features have been ascribed to the peculiar anatomy and physiology of some areas of the body (although this is speculative, because only a minority of nevi from sites recognized as "special" do show a true site-related atypia) [7,40].

- Of paramount importance for the recognition of these lesions as benign is the clinicopathological correlation, inasmuch as most nevi with site-related atypia are relatively small (with the exception of congenital nevi) and excised in young patients because of a clinical atypia that is usually not so striking as to clinically favor melanoma.
- *Genital nevi* in young women may show a high degree of melanocytic atypia both within the epidermis (upward extension, deep adnexal extension, irregular confluence of nests, and/or lentiginous proliferation) and within the superficial dermis (confluent growth of epithelioid and/or spindle melanocytes); however, maturation is readily appreciated and mitotic activity is absent [41]. In addition, it must be underlined that, different from atypical genital nevi, melanoma of the vulva is almost invariably diagnosed in the elderly [42].
- *Atypical acral nevi* can show a prevailingly lentiginous pattern [43], but vertically oriented nests are invariably seen and often predominate. Focal pagetoid extension is commonly present, particularly toward the center; lesions with striking upward migration (about 60% of cases) have been described as melanocytic acral nevi with intraepidermal ascent of cells (M.A.N.I.A.C.s) [44]. However, in such tumors, cells are epithelioid (rather than spindle) and remarkably monomorphic; in addition, acanthosis is mild and regular, there is no lymphocytic infiltrate, and the dermal component, if present, invariably looks bland. Mild fibrosis may be seen particularly in nevi of the sole and this is often misconstrued as evidence of "dysplasia" or even regression. Fig. 7.1.5 outlines an example of M.A.N.I.A.C.s underlining the importance of the clinicopathological correlation.
- *Atypical nevi of the scalp* are most commonly found in adolescents [45] and clinically display central tan or pink coloration with a darker peripheral rim ("eclipse nevi") [46]. Histopathologically, the growth pattern may be "dysplastic nevus-like" (bridging of the junctional nests and exaggerated lamellar fibrosis) or "superficial congenital nevus-like" (large junctional nests both at the tips and at the sides of the rete ridges; common involvement of the adnexa). Upward migration of melanocytes in the central part of the lesion, lentiginous proliferation, dermal nests larger than the junctional nests, and a few dermal mitoses may be disturbing architectural features. In our experience, some features of atypical nevi of the scalp recall a sclerosing nevus with pseudomelanomatus features. The young age of the patients, the prevailing nested growth pattern, the lack of relevant cytologic atypia, and the preserved maturation pattern are the main differential features from melanoma.
- *Atypical melanocytic nevi of the ankle* are most commonly found in young to middle-aged women: the architectural disorder can be severe, with a prevailingly single cell proliferation, lack of

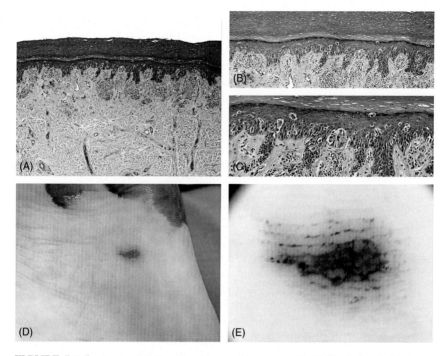

FIGURE 7.1.5   **An acral lesion in a 44-year-old woman.** (A–C) The lesion is thin compound with a bland-appearing dermal component. There is a slightly irregular epidermal hyperplasia with several melanocytes in single units and small nests within the upper layer of the epidermis. (D) Clinically, the lesion is medium-sized and asymmetric. (E) Dermoscopy shows that the periphery of the lesion is characterized by a parallel furrow pattern that is typical for acral nevi. Thus, the lesion is clinically atypical but not enough to think of melanoma: this is the common scenario of nevi in special sites. Histopathological diagnosis: melanocytic acral nevus with intraepidermal ascent of cells (M.A.N.I.A.C.s).

circumscription, and melanin within the stratum corneum; typically, however, cytologic atypia is only mild to moderate; different from dysplastic nevi, there is no dermal fibroplasia [47].

- *Flexural melanocytic nevi* may show great variability in the size of junctional nests, with some of them placed at the sides of the rete ridges; large dermal nests may even predominate, but maturation is well preserved, cytologic atypia is mild, and mitotic figures are not observed [48]. Dermal fibrosis is horizontal and compact, rather than concentric/lamellar like in dysplastic nevi. The overall picture can resemble genital nevi.
- *Breast/milk line nevi* are usually removed in patients younger than 35 years with no sex predilection. Two histopathological patterns can be recognized: (1) nested, with a typical "garland-like" confluence of junctional nests of large and pale melanocytes; (2) lentiginous,

with a prevailing single cell proliferation at the junction, poor lateral circumscription, and hyperpigmentation/transepidermal melanin elimination. The latter pattern predominates on the nipple and areola [40,49]. In both variants, widespread cytologic atypia and mitotic activity are not features; stromal response is variable.

- *Nevi occurring on and around the ear* can show atypical features including asymmetry, poor circumscription, some pagetoid scatter, and even severe cytologic atypia (junctional and dermal melanocytes with epithelioid morphology, prominent vesicular nuclei, a single basophilic nucleolus, and pink cytoplasm). Nevertheless, the lesions are commonly small, with a preserved maturation pattern and no mitotic activity [50,51].

- *Nevi of the conjunctiva* are almost invariably atypical in their junctional component, which is typified by a prevailingly lentiginous growth and some horizontally oriented nests; the epithelium is thin and contains mucus-secreting cells that may be mistaken for pagetoid cells. However, these nevi are usually small and, if compound, show a very bland lymphocyte-like dermal component that is associated with epithelial cysts and pseudoglandular spaces: these are unique to this site and virtually diagnostic of benignity [40,52].

- Nevi in special sites are a good example of the impossibility to predict the risk of evolution into melanoma of a nevus on the basis of its histopathological features: in fact, these nevi can be even severely atypical, but melanoma in special sites is only exceptionally associated with a nevus [1]. In other words, an "intermediate" morphology does not necessarily imply an "intermediate" biology.

- In conclusion, in many—or most—instances, the "gray zone" in melanocytic skin neoplasms is "subjective," inasmuch as it reflects a diagnostic, rather than a truly biological problem: under this circumstance, a lesion can be labeled with items such as "superficial atypical melanocytic proliferation of uncertain significance" (S.A.M.P.U.S.) if intraepidermal or thin compound; or "melanocytic tumor of uncertain malignant potential" (MEL.T.U.M.P.) if thick compound or dermal-based [53].

- We warn that the use of the diagnostic label "dysplastic nevus" for a lesion with conflicting histopathological features can be strongly misleading.

3 MELANOCYTIC NEOPLASMS WITH UNPREDICTABLE BIOLOGICAL BEHAVIOR

- Besides the relatively common scenario of melanocytic skin neoplasms with conflicting histopathological features, there is a small subset of melanocytic skin neoplasms that are "biologically intermediate" inasmuch as they are capable of involvement of regional lymph nodes but have limited potential for distant spread [3,54,55].

- The term melanocytoma has been recently proposed for this group of lesions, with a nevus/melanocytoma/melanoma classification scheme that is aimed at reflecting the existence of a true "morphobiological spectrum" ranging from benignity to full-blown malignancy [55].
  - The main candidates for the inclusion into the "melanocytoma" rubric are as follows:
    - (Atypical) Spitz tumor
    - Atypical dermal dendritic melanocytic proliferations (also referred to as "pigmented epithelioid melanocytoma" and including epithelioid blue nevus and animal-type melanoma) [35]
    - Atypical deep penetrating nevus/deep penetrating-like borderline melanocytic tumor [56]
- It must be underlined that MEL.T.U.M.P. and melanocytoma are not synonyms (Table 7.1.6): in fact, the former is a merely descriptive term defining a diagnostic uncertainty, whereas the latter identifies a morphologically distinct subset of melanocytic tumors whose biological properties are in keeping with the hypothesis of a low-grade (lymphotropic) malignancy. In our view, there is little doubt that in a dichotomic (nevus vs. melanoma) diagnostic approach, most if not all melanocytomas should

TABLE 7.1.6   Comparison of the Definitional Features for Melanocytic Tumors of Uncertain Malignant Potential (MEL.T.U.M.P.) and Melanocytoma

	MEL.T.U.M.P	Melanocytoma
Definition	Broad morphological spectrum of melanocytic tumors in vertical growth phase (nevi with severe atypia, melanocytomas, deceptively bland melanomas)	Dermal-based neoplasm, often with little involvement of the epidermis
Specific diagnostic criteria	None	Identifiable
Genetics	Possibly similar to "conventional" melanoma	Growing number of specific alterations
Behavior	If malignant, possibly similar to "conventional" melanoma	Frequent regional involvement; rare distant metastases
Proposed management	As per conventional melanoma	Wide local excision plus echotomographic monitoring of the regional nodes

be labeled as "melanoma" and that the nodal involvement of melanocytoma should be considered as "metastasis." However, the biological potential of melanocytomas is completely different from that of "conventional" melanoma; thus, these neoplasms probably require treatment and follow-up protocols that are conceivably different from those required by "conventional" melanoma. The main problem with this approach is that it should be validated with a long clinical follow-up of sufficient number of cases, and, since melanocytomas are quite unusual lesions, such a goal is not easy to be achieved [1].

3.1 (Atypical) Spitz Tumor

- Dermal-based melanocytic proliferation that shows architectural and cytological (predominance of large epithelioid and/or spindle cells) features recalling a Spitz nevus but is "tumorigenic":
  - That is, characterized by a nodular silhouette made by confluent sheets of cells in the dermis without intervening collagen, and/or by a (nontraumatic) ulceration, and/or by a relevant mitotic activity (more than occasional mitotic figures and/or mitoses close to the base) and/or confluent (nonrandom) pleomorphism [23,26]
- The term "atypical" may be redundant because, if classified as "tumorigenic," a spitzoid neoplasm is implicitly "atypical."
- Table 7.1.7 illustrates the differential features between "atypical Spitz nevus" and "(atypical) Spitz tumor" [23,26].
- The average rate of sentinel node positivity in (atypical) Spitz tumors is 38%–39% [57,58]; instead, distant metastases are rare, especially in prepubescent patients [58]. In Fig. 7.1.6 is an atypical Spitz tumor with sentinel node involvement.
- The recognition of cases of atypical Spitz tumor with fatal outcome can prove impossible on morphological grounds alone [3]; molecular techniques are currently under investigation regarding their potential to help prognosticate these tumors [59–62].

3.2 Atypical Dermal Dendritic Melanocytic Proliferations

- The term "melanocytoma" derives from an extension of the concept of *pigmented epithelioid melanocytoma*; this was proposed in 2004 for a low-grade melanocytic malignancy (nodal involvement in 46% of cases but no disease-related death) showing overlapping features between an atypical epithelioid blue nevus and a low-grade "animal-type (equine-type) melanoma" (or "pigment-synthesizing melanoma" or "dendritic cell melanoma") [35,36,63].

TABLE 7.1.7   Proposed Histopathological Criteria for the Differential Diagnosis Between Atypical Spitz Nevus and Spitz Tumor

Microscopic features	Atypical Spitz nevus	(Atypical) Spitz tumor
Size (mm)	7–10	>10
Tumorigenicity (nodule)	−	+
Asymmetry	Superficial	Deep +/− superficial
Sharp circumscription, intraepidermal	+/−	+/−
Sharp circumscription, lateral dermal	−	−/+
Sharp circumscription, deep dermal	−	+/++
Epidermal atrophy	−/+	+/++
Ulceration	−	−/+
Large dermal nests	Superficial	Deep +/− superficial
Dermal sheets of cells	−	+/++
Deep extension	−	+
Melanin in the depth	−	−/+
Cytologic atypia	Focal ("random")	Widespread
Maturation	+	−
Mitotic figures	Few	Numerous, in crops, and/or close to the base

- Epithelioid blue nevus was first described in Carney's complex [64], a familial lentiginosis with a low-grade multiorgan neoplasia (Table 7.1.8) due to mutations in the PRKAR1A gene (OMIM 188830) coding for the regulatory subunit type I alpha of the protein kinase A [65]. After a seminal paper by Carney and Ferreiro [64], sporadic cases of epithelioid blue nevus have been increasingly reported [35]. Both syndromic and sporadic epithelioid blue nevi are typified as small- to medium-sized, wedge-shaped tumors with hyperplastic, normal, or atrophic epidermis and no appreciable grenz zone; the dermal-based proliferation is made by an admixture of heavily pigmented small epithelioid cells, nonpigmented (or less heavily pigmented) large epithelioid cells, and dendritic melanocytes; mitotic activity and necrosis are consistently absent [35].

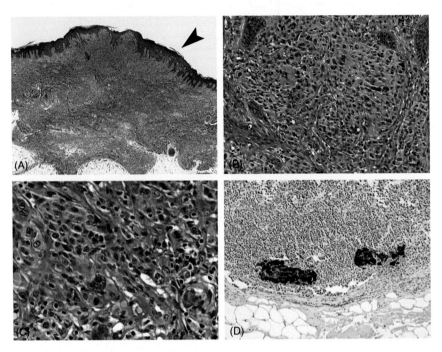

FIGURE 7.1.6 **A spitzoid melanocytic tumor removed from the thigh of a 7-year-old boy.** (A) The tumor is wedge-shaped but with a clearly asymmetric epidermal involvement (*arrow*). (B) The dermal nests are irregularly confluent. (C) There is also confluent cytological pleomorphism with random melanin synthesis. (D) Sentinel node biopsy showing multiple subcapsular aggregates of S100-positive melanocytes. Histopathological diagnosis: atypical Spitz tumor with sentinel node involvement. Completion lymph node dissection was not performed. The patient is alive with no evidence of disease after 9 years.

- On the opposite end of the morphobiological spectrum is animal-type melanoma, a rare subtype of melanoma closely resembling the heavily pigmented melanocytic tumors found in gray horses older than 15 years [66]. In humans, animal-type melanoma occurs in young to middle-aged individuals; the scalp is a common location; even being very often a thick tumor with frequent involvement of the sentinel node, its prognosis seems to be much better than a "conventional" melanoma of the same thickness [67].
- Histological features favoring malignancy in an epithelioid and dendritic cell neoplasm are the following:
  - Large size
  - Asymmetric involvement of the epidermis
  - Ulceration
  - Quadrangular shape
  - Mitotic activity (>2 mitoses/mmq)

TABLE 7.1.8 Diagnostic Criteria for Carney's Complex[a]

MAJOR CRITERIA

1. Spotty skin pigmentation with typical distribution (lips, conjunctiva and inner or outer canthi, vaginal and penile mucosal)
2. Myxoma[b] (cutaneous and mucosal) or cardiac myxoma[b]
3. Breast myxomatosis[b] or fat-suppressed magnetic resonance imaging findings suggestive of this diagnosis
4. Primary pigmented nodular adrenocortical disease[b] or paradoxical positive response of urinary glucocorticosteroid excretion to dexamethasone administration during Liddle's test
5. Acromegaly as a result of growth hormone–producing adenoma
6. Large-cell calcifying Sertoli cell tumor[b] or characteristic calcification on testicular ultrasound
7. Thyroid carcinoma (at any age) or multiple hypoechoic nodules on thyroid ultrasound in prepubertal child
8. Psammomatous melanotic schwannomas[b]
9. Blue nevus, epithelioid blue nevus (multiple)[b]
10. Breast ductal adenoma (multiple)[b]
11. Osteochondromyxoma[b]

SUPPLEMENTAL CRITERIA

1. Affected first-degree relative
2. Activating pathogenic variants of PRKACA (single base substitutions and copy number variation) and PRKACB
3. Inactivating mutation of the PRKAR1A gene

MINOR CRITERIA

1. Intense freckling (without darkly pigmented spots or typical distribution)
2. Blue nevus, common type (if multiple)
3. Café-au-lait spots or other "birthmarks"
4. Elevated IGFI levels, abnormal glucose tolerance test, or paradoxical GH response to thyrotropin-releasing hormone testing in the absence of clinical acromegaly
5. Cardiomyopathy
6. History of Cushing's syndrome, acromegaly, or sudden death in extended family
7. Pilonidal sinus
8. Colonic polyps (usually in association with acromegaly)
9. Multiple skin tags or other skin lesions; lipomas
10. Hyperprolactinemia (usually mild and almost always combined with clinical or subclinical acromegaly)
11. Single, benign thyroid nodule in a child younger than age 18 years; multiple thyroid nodules in an individual older than age 18 years (detected on ultrasound examination)
12. Family history of carcinoma, in particular of the thyroid, colon, pancreas, and ovary; other multiple benign or malignant tumors

[a]*To make the diagnosis of CNC, a patient must either (1) exhibit two of the major criteria confirmed by histology, imaging, or biochemical testing or (2) meet one major criterion and one supplemental one. Minor criteria can only suggest further investigation.*
[b]*With histological confirmation.*

- Inflammation
- Necrosis
- Nonrandom (confluent) atypia of the epithelioid component
- Dendritic cells with thick and irregular processes
  - We cautiously suggest that even the presence of only one of these features may be not compatible with benignity: intuitively, however, the final evaluation depends on the quantitative representation of each of these criteria of "atypia," thereby justifying the adoption of the "pigmented epithelioid melanocytoma" category for a broad gray zone in the middle of the spectrum [68].

3.3 Atypical Deep Penetrating Nevus and Deep Penetrating-Like Borderline Melanocytic Tumor

- Deep penetrating nevus is characterized by wedge shape, sharp circumscription, and vertical orientation along the adnexa and the neurovascular bundles [69–71]; the tumor is composed of epithelioid (type A) cells with "dusty" melanin, sometimes with a multivacuolated cytoplasm (sebocyte-like cells) [34], and/or by pale spindle (type C) cells; characteristically, these cells are arranged in small nests with the intervening stroma infiltrated by dendritic melanocytes and melanophages in a very tidy fashion ("checkerboard" pattern of pigment distribution); pleomorphism can be striking, but it is usually "random" (nonconfluent); mitotic figures are absent or sparse. As well recognized since 1992 [70], the typical reassuring morphological context is a combined nevus in which the deep penetrating component is not predominant.
- Size >1 cm, quadrangular/horizontal/nodular silhouette, asymmetry, inflammation, and mitotic figures >2 mmq^{-1} are worrisome features: in our opinion, outside the "combined" context, even one of these features is enough to label the tumor as "atypical" or "borderline" (Fig. 7.1.7). In the presence of "atypical" features, the percentage of sentinel node involvement is about 33% [35].

4 THE "GRAY ZONE" AND THE ANCILLARY TECHNIQUES

The bulk of the "gray zone" issue has prompted pathologists to look for new weapons in their diagnostic armamentarium for melanocytic skin neoplasms.

- Immunohistochemistry is the most widely adopted ancillary technique. As already underlined in Chapter 3.4, an acceptable

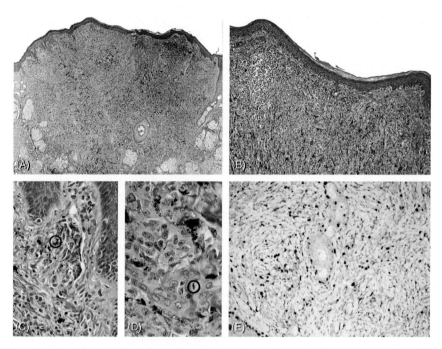

FIGURE 7.1.7   **A dermal-based spindle cell melanocytic tumor removed from the nose in a 19-year-old man.** (A) The lesion is vaguely wedge-shaped but clearly asymmetric and inflamed. (B) There is a sparse and asymmetric junctional component. (C and D) Mitoses are easily found (*circles*). (E) The Ki67 labeling of tumor cells is higher than expected for a fully benign lesion. Histopathological diagnosis: deep penetrating-like borderline melanocytic tumor.

compromise between cost, increase in technical routine workload, and diagnostic information can be achieved with the adoption of a panel composed of the antibodies against: (1) the cell cycle–related protein Ki67; (2) the human melanoma black (HMB) 45; (3) the p16 protein. A "clustered" and/or high (>13%) Ki67 labeling, an abnormal HMB45 staining pattern (lack of a "maturation" pattern; focal loss of reactivity in dermal dendritic melanocytic proliferations), and an "untidy" p16 immunoreactivity (complete negativity or confluent areas of negativity) are worrisome features [72]. Unfortunately, however, not any single immunostain is able to give clear-cut information for the differential diagnosis; moreover, the interpretation of the immunohistochemical results is often very subjective itself.
• The use of comparative genomic hybridization (CGH) to detect the genome-wide DNA copy number changes in solid tumors has been revolutionary given that the technique can be performed on routinely processed tissue samples. The copy number change needs to be present in about 30%–50% of the cells in order to be identifiable, depending on

the type of aberration [73,74]. In contrast, array CGH allows for a more accurate quantification of DNA copy number and reliable detection of single-copy deletions or duplications, thereby improving resolution [74,75]. The observation of frequent chromosomal aberrations in melanoma and a relative absence of aberrations in melanocytic nevi suggest that chromosomal analysis could be exploited diagnostically in ambiguous melanoctic tumors, including spitzoid melanocytic neoplasms [76–78]. Several studies have now shown that chromosomal copy number aberrations involving a variety of loci are typical of melanoma while Spitz nevi are associated with only a limited variety of copy number aberrations, including gains of 11p in the HRAS locus and much more rarely 7q [79–82]. Gains involving 11p are specifically found in some spitzoid tumors (compound or dermal "V"-shaped proliferations with deep desmoplasia), also known as "HRASomas" or "Bastian nevi" [79]: with only rare exceptions [83], such findings are a hallmark of benignity.

- Mutation analysis is mostly useful for the differential diagnosis between melanocytic tumors belonging to different morphological categories. For example, spitzoid and dermal dendritic melanocytic proliferations usually do not harbor BRAF/NRAS mutations; thus, if such an occurrence is documented, a careful morphological reevaluation is warranted in order to rule out a "conventional" melanocytic malignancy. In addition, it has been recently suggested that hTERT promoter activating mutations can be associated with an aggressive behavior of atypical Spitz tumors, even if the number of tested cases with fatal outcome to date is very low [84].
- In recent years fluorescence in situ hybridization (FISH) has been increasingly used for morphologically challenging cases. The standard melanoma FISH test targeting RREB1 (6p25), MYB (6q23), CCND1 (11q13), and centromere 6 was set up on the basis of CGH studies as an effective compromise between cost, technical complexity, and sensitivity [85,86]. We currently use the standard FISH positivity as a tiebreaker for challenging melanocytic neoplasms mainly in a nonspitzoid morphological context, because the currently available test leaves several unresolved issues, namely:
  - A relatively low diagnostic accuracy in morphologically ambiguous melanocytic neoplasms
  - A relatively low sensitivity and specificity in spitzoid neoplasms
  - The occurrence of false-positives due to tetraploidy in Spitz nevi and in nevi with an atypical epithelioid component [87]
    - Under investigation is a new melanoma probe cocktail targeting RREB1 (6p25), C-MYC (8q24), CDKN2A (9p21), and CCND1 (11q13) [88,89]. However, the new melanoma probe

cocktail has been tested on very few cases of atypical spitzoid proliferations with fatal outcome and this prevents any clear-cut conclusion. For all the earlier discussion, we have proposed the implementation of a FISH algorithm (standard four-probe test followed by either C-MYC or CDKN2A/centromere 9) [87] as shown in Fig. 7.1.8: of note is the pivotal role of the clinical information, as well as of the overall morphological context.

Using break-apart FISH probes Wiesner et al. [90] have also described spitzoid neoplasms with kinase fusions of *ROS1* (17%), *NTRK1* (16%), *ALK* (10%), *BRAF* (5%), and *RET* (3%); these alterations are present along the entire spectrum of spitzoid tumors (55% of Spitz nevi; 56% of atypical Spitz tumors; 39% of spitzoid melanomas). Neoplasms with fusion of ALK (with either tropomyosin 3 or dynactin 1 as fusion partners) are typically polypoid with a plexiform (fascicular) growth of spindle-shaped melanocytes [25]: these tumors seem to behave in a benign fashion (Dr. Thomas Wiesner, personal communication), even if follow-up data are relatively limited to date.

- In conclusion, clear-cut diagnostic information from the ancillary techniques can be expected in a very limited number of morphologically/morphobiologically ambiguous melanocytic proliferations. Moreover, with the relevant exception of immunohistochemistry, these techniques are laborious and expensive and require highly specialized personnel and equipment: thus, their applicability is limited to highly qualified and specialized centers.

5 PATHOLOGICAL HANDLING AND REPORTING

- The histopathological report must include all the pertinent clinical information and a thorough macroscopic description comprising the sampling protocol adopted.
- It has been demonstrated that full clinical information, comprising the clinical pictures, can increase the histopathologists' "confidence" in their diagnosis [91,92]. In addition, the clinicodermoscopic features of any pigmented skin tumor can be used as a guide to the gross sampling of respective excision specimen [21]: ex vivo examination with a cross-polarized light dermatoscope followed by marking of the area(s) of interest with nail varnish has been proposed to secure a histopathological examination targeted to the clinically suspicious areas of any skin tumor [93]. Nevertheless, such techniques are time-consuming and must be implemented by histopathologists with specific expertise in clinical dermatology and dermoscopy: thus,

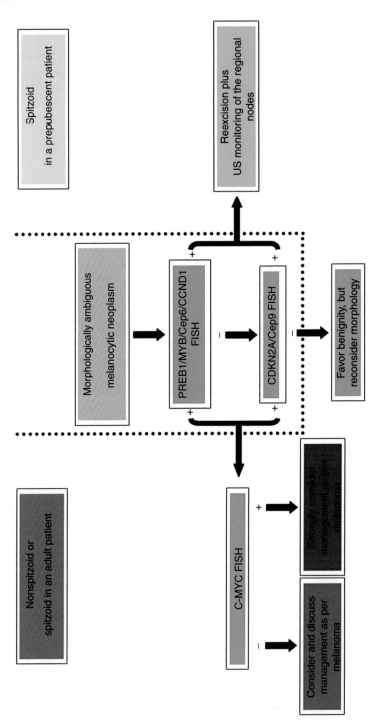

FIGURE 7.1.8 The algorithm proposed for the evaluation of morphologically ambiguous melanocytic tumors with fluorescence in situ hybridization. Note the pivotal role of the clinical data.

only a few selected cases will be finally handled according to careful protocols of clinicopathological correlation.

- As a complementary/alternative method, after any histopathological report is rendered, the clinician can review the respective case in light of the clinical–dermoscopic pictures; cases for which a good clinicopathological correlation is missing are reviewed in a multidisciplinary team meeting by the referral clinicians and the referral dermatopathologist in order to achieve a consensus on the final diagnosis and the management (see the subsequent text) [94].
- In the presence of any diagnostic uncertainty, the minimal requirements of the histopathological report are suggested to be the following:
  - A careful microscopic description underlining the "conflicting" morphological criteria of the case. This is a highly technical section of the report [95] that must reflect the thoroughness of the histological study performed and represents the basis of the histopathological diagnosis and its uncertainty.
  - A "provisional diagnosis" (better referred to as a "diagnostic proposal") according to a terminology that should mirror the elements of doubts. We suggest the following diagnostic categories:
    - *Atypical (junctional/compound/dermal) melanocytic nevus*, for a neoplasm that is felt to be most likely benign.
    - *Severely atypical (junctional/thin compound/thick compound/ dermal based) melanocytic proliferation (with features of ___)* for a neoplasm that is possibly/probably malignant.
    - As an alternative, the "severely atypical" category can be labeled with the acronyms S.A.M.P.U.S. and MEL.T.U.M.P. [53] for melanocytic neoplasms that are intraepidermal/ thin compound and thick compound/dermal, respectively. A "thick compound" melanocytic neoplasm is defined on the basis of the criteria for vertical growth phase melanoma (see Chapter 3.4).
  - A statement about the internal (intradepartmental) consultation(s) achieved because of the conflicting morphological features of the case. Even if the diagnosis finally remains controversial, an explicit statement about intradepartmental consultation(s) is suggested for medicolegal reasons.
  - An indication to the management. An in toto excision with clear margins must be requested for any atypical melanocytic proliferation that has been incompletely excised or submitted to incision biopsy (see the subsequent text). Any further decision about the management and the follow-up should be explicitly referred to a discussion in an ad hoc multidisciplinary team meeting.

- Optional diagnostic evaluations and parameters to be considered for inclusion in the histopathological report are the following:
  - The assignment of a given melanocytic proliferation to a specific subgroup of neoplasms (e.g., spitzoid, dermal dendritic cell). Even if ad hoc formal studies are still lacking, in our experience such an assignment is often a matter of sizable disagreement by itself.
  - Ancillary techniques (immunohistochemical and molecular biology). It has been demonstrated that an expert diagnosis is not changed by the results of immunohistochemical and molecular techniques, even in the setting of morphologically controversial melanocytic tumors [96]. Thus, these data cannot be considered as a sine qua non for the diagnostic evaluation.
  - External expert consultation. Even experts consistently disagree on the morphological diagnosis of melanocytic lesions [3,33,91,92,97]. Thus, an expert consultation is far from being a statement of absolute truth; moreover, it is not easy and fast to be achieved all over the world. This is why, even if desirable, it cannot be considered as compulsory. Even more important, an expert consultation cannot replace a multidisciplinary team-based evaluation.

6 GUIDELINES FOR MANAGEMENT

- Every surgical procedure resulting in an incomplete removal of a histopathologically atypical melanocytic neoplasm must be followed by a reexcision with clear margins.
- A histopathological diagnosis of "atypical nevus" implies a clinical reevaluation aimed at individuating clinical/environmental modifiers (ultraviolet exposure, drugs, trauma, epilation) that might explain some histopathological features of atypia; in addition, the surgical scar should be monitored and every recurrent lesion should be promptly excised and sent to the histopathologist with the request for reevaluation of the slides from the previous excision specimen.
- A narrow reexcision is advised for atypical Spitz nevi [26] and atypical blue nevi because their boundary with the respective "melanocytomas" is blurred.
- All "melanocytomas" should undergo adequate reexcision (the extent of which also depends on the resulting aesthetic/functional impairment); instead, the decision about performing sentinel node biopsy should be made by preliminarily considering that in these

tumors the finding of isolated tumor cells in the sentinel node is not an unequivocal sign of "conventional" melanocytic malignancy (i.e., melanoma) [98,99] and is not an indication to completion lymphadenectomy, based on the ambiguity of the primary. It must be also underlined that, in a recent metaanalysis, 98%–99% of young patients with Spitz tumors had no evidence of disease after a median follow-up of 59 months, regardless of the sentinel node positivity [58]: therefore the diagnostic and prognostic information given by a positive sentinel node in young patients seems to be negligible. An echotomographic monitoring of the regional nodes (and an echotomography-guided fine needle aspiration biopsy cytology) can even replace sentinel node biopsy, because it allows to efficiently detect massive replacement of the node(s) by neoplastic cells, thereby addressing selected patients to election lymphadenectomy [99]. Such a follow-up protocol is probably the best choice in patients younger than 10 years, especially for lesions located in the head/neck area, a region in which surgical procedures are aesthetically relevant and are hampered by a sizable failure rate [100].

- The final decision about the management should be set up by means of a multidisciplinary team discussion; every option should be discussed with the patients or their guardians in order to implement a strategy on an informed consent basis.
- Pathology review may be requested for patients when care is transferred to a tertiary care referral center: if it is true that this practice has many benefits, unforeseen difficulties in doctor–patient communication and even medicolegal problems may be raised, especially when a diagnosis is changed after some or many years [101]. No guidelines exist to date for pathology reviews. We suggest that:
  - The original H&E-stained slides should be always examined.
  - Since the microscopic picture can substantially change with histological recuts, the review report should always consider at first the microscopic features as found in the original slides.
  - The original diagnosis should be always carefully discussed within a thorough microscopic description, especially if the diagnosis has to be overturned or modified.
  - Additional immunohistochemical and molecular investigation performed should be detailed along with their practical impact on the final diagnosis.
  - A feedback to the secondary care center should be promptly given in any case (irrespective of the final diagnosis of the pathology review).

7 CONCLUSIONS

The "gray zone" in the histopathological diagnosis of melanocytic skin is a matter of fact in daily practice. In recent years, both melanocytic neoplasms with intermediate morphology (atypical nevi and morphologically bland melanomas) and melanocytic neoplasms with intermediate biology (melanocytic tumors with a high rate of nodal involvement but a very low rate of distant metastases) have been thoroughly investigated with molecular techniques, but clear-cut results impacting on patients' management are still far to be achieved. The original reports, the expert consultations, and the pathology reviews should carefully underline the diagnostic challenges of any single case. The management of these neoplasms should be decided on an informed consent basis; any proposals about the management should be delivered with a multidisciplinary team approach.

References

[1] Ferrara G, Senetta R, Paglierani M, Massi D. Main clues in the pathological diagnosis of melanoma: is molecular genetics helping? Dermatol Ther 2012;25:423–31.

[2] Ackerman AB. Malignant melanoma: a unifying concept. Hum Pathol 1980;11:591–5.

[3] Cerroni L, Barnhill R, Elder D, Gottlieb G, Heenan P, Kutzner H, et al. Melanocytic tumors of uncertain malignant potential: results of a tutorial held at the XXIX Symposium of the International Society of Dermatopathology in Graz, October 2008. Am J Surg Pathol 2010;34:314–26.

[4] Harbst K, Staaf J, Lauss M, Karlsson A, Måsbäck A, Johansson I, et al. Molecular profiling reveals low- and high-grade forms of primary melanoma. Clin Cancer Res 2012;18:4026–36.

[5] Magro CM, Crowson AN, Mihm MC, Kline M. De novo intraepidermal epithelioid melanocytic dysplasia: an emerging entity. J Cutan Pathol 2010;37:866–9.

[6] Kim JC, Murphy GF. Dysplastic melanocytic nevi and prognostically indeterminate nevomelanomatoid proliferations. Clin Lab Med 2000;20:691–712.

[7] Cook DL. Melanocytic naevi of special sites. Diagn Histopathol 2010;16(7):309–16.

[8] Glatz K, Hartmann C, Antic M, Kutzner H. Frequent mitotic activity in banal melanocytic nevi uncovered by immunohistochemical analysis. Am J Dermatopathol 2010;32:643–9.

[9] Kokta V, Hung T, Al Dhaybi R, Lugassy C, Barnhill RL. High prevalence of angiotropism in congenital melanocytic nevi: an analysis of 53 cases. Am J Dermatopathol 2013;35:180.

[10] Urso C. A new perspective for Spitz tumors? Am J Dermatopathol 2005;27:364–7.

[11] Kerl H, Soyer HP, Cerroni L, Wolf IH, Ackerman AB. Ancient melanocytic nevus. Semin Diagn Pathol 1998;15:210–5.

[12] Clark WH Jr, Reimer RR, Greene M, Ainsworth AM, Mastrangelo MJ. Origin of familial malignant melanomas from heritable melanocytic lesions. Arch Dermatol 1978;114:732–8.

[13] Elder DE, Goldman LI, Goldman SC, Greene MH, Cark WH Jr. Dysplastic nevus syndrome: a phenotypic association of sporadic cutaneous melanoma. Cancer 1980;46:1787–94.

[14] Cockerel CJ, Grant-Kels J, Cather JC, LeBoit PE. Dysplastic nevus. In: Le Boit PE, Burg G, Weedon D, Sarasin A, editors. World Health Organization classification of tumours—pathology and genetics of skin tumours. Lyon: IARC Press; 2006. p. 105–9.

[15] Kaddu S, Smolle J, Zenahlik P, Hofmann-Wellenhof R, Kerl H. Melanoma with benign melanocytic naevus components: reappraisal of clinicopathological features and prognosis. Melanoma Res 2002;12:271–8.

[16] Fox JC, Reed JA, Shea CR. The recurrent nevus phenomenon: a history of challenge, controversy, and discovery. Arch Pathol Lab Med 2011;135:842–6.

[17] Fabrizi G, Pennacchia I, Pagliarello C, Massi G. Sclerosing nevus with pseudomelanomatous features. J Cutan Pathol 2008;35:995–1002.

[18] Ferrara G, Amantea A, Argenziano G, Broganelli P, Cesinaro AM, Donati P, et al. Sclerosing nevus with pseudomelanomatous features and regressing melanoma with nevoid features. J Cutan Pathol 2009;36:913–5.

[19] Ferrara G, Giorgio CM, Zalaudek I, Broganelli P, Pellacani G, Tomasini C, et al. Sclerosing nevus with pseudomelanomatous features (nevus with regression-like fibrosis): clinical and dermoscopic features of a recently characterized histopathologic entity. Dermatology 2009;219:202–8.

[20] Ko CJ, Bolognia JL, Glusac EJ. "Clark/dysplastic" nevi with florid fibroplasia associated with pseudomelanomatous features. J Am Acad Dermatol 2011;64:346–51.

[21] Ferrara G, Argenziano G, Giorgio CM, Zalaudek I, Kittler H. Dermoscopic–pathologic correlation: apropos of six equivocal cases. Semin Cutan Med Surg 2009;28:157–64.

[22] Suh KY, Bolognia JL. Signature nevi. J Am Acad Dermatol 2009;60:508–14.

[23] Ferrara G, Gianotti R, Cavicchini S, Salviato T, Zalaudek I, Argenziano G. Spitz nevus, Spitz tumor and spitzoid melanoma: a comprehensive clinicopathologic overview. Dermatol Clin 2013;31:589–98. viii.

[24] Argenziano G, Zalaudek I, Ferrara G, Lorenzoni A, Soyer HP. Involution: the natural evolution of pigmented Spitz and Reed nevi? Arch Dermatol 2007;143:549–51.

[25] Busam K, Kutzner H, Cerroni L, Wiesner T. Clinical and pathologic findings of Spitz nevi and atypical Spitz tumors with ALK fusions. Am J Surg Pathol 2014;38:925–33.

[26] Ferrara G, Cavicchini S, Corradin MT. Hypopigmented atypical spitzoid neoplasms (atypical Spitz nevi, atypical Spitz tumors, spitzoid melanoma): a clinicopathological update. Dermatol Pract Concept 2015;5:45–52.

[27] Wiesner T, Obenauf AC, Murali R, Fried I, Griewank KG, Ulz P, et al. Germline mutations in BAP1 predispose to melanocytic tumors. Nat Genet 2011;43:1018–21.

[28] Njauw CN, Kim I, Piris A, Gabree M, Taylor M, Lane AM, et al. Germline BAP1 inactivation is preferentially associated with metastatic ocular melanoma and cutaneous-ocular melanoma families. PLoS One 2012;7:e35295.

[29] Wiesner T, Murali R, Fried I, Cerroni L, Busam K, Kutzner H, et al. A distinct subset of atypical Spitz tumors is characterized by BRAF mutation and loss of BAP1 expression. Am J Surg Pathol 2012;36:818–30.

[30] Yeh I, Mully TW, Wieser T, Vemula SS, Mirza SA, Sparatta AJ, et al. Ambiguous melanocytic tumors with loss of 3p21. Am J Surg Pathol 2014;38:1088–95.

[31] Piris A, Mihm MC Jr, Hoang MP. BAP1 and BRAFV600E expression in benign and malignant melanocytic proliferations. Hum Pathol 2015;46:239–45.

[32] Vilain RE, McCarthy SW, Thompson JF, Scolyer RA. BAP1-inactivated spitzoid naevi. Am J Surg Pathol 2015;39:722.

[33] Barnhill RL, Argenyi Z, Berwick M, Duray PH, Erickson L, Guitart J, et al. Atypical cellular blue nevi (cellular blue nevi with atypical features): lack of consensus for diagnosis and distinction from cellular blue nevi and malignant melanoma ("malignant blue nevus"). Am J Surg Pathol 2008;32:36–44.

[34] Ferrara G, Soyer HP, Malvehy J, Piccolo D, Puig S, Sopena J, et al. The many faces of blue nevus: a clinicopathologic study. J Cutan Pathol 2007;34:543–51.

[35] Zembowicz A, Mihm MC. Dermal dendritic melanocytic proliferations: an update. Histopathology 2004;45:433–51.

[36] Nicholls DS, Mason GH. Halo dermatitis around a melanocytic naevus: Meyerson's naevus. Br J Dermatol 1988;118:125–9.

[37] Rodins K, Byrom L, Muir J. Early melanoma with halo eczema (Meyerson's phenomenon). Australas J Dermatol 2011;52:70–3.

[38] Pižem J, Stojanovič L, Luzar B. Melanocytic lesions with eczematous reaction (Meyerson's phenomenon)—a histopathologic analysis of 64 cases. J Cutan Pathol 2012;39:901–10.

[39] ElShabrawi-Caelen L, Soyer HP, Schaeppi H, Cerroni L, Schirren CG, Rudolph C, et al. Genital lentigines and melanocytic nevi with superimposed lichen sclerosus: a diagnostic challenge. J Am Acad Dermatol 2004;50:690–4.

[40] Hosler GA, Moresi JM, Barrett TL. Nevi with site-related atypia: a review of melanocytic nevi with atypical histologic features based on anatomic site. J Cutan Pathol 2008;35:889–98.

[41] Ribé A. Melanocytic lesions of the genital area with attention given to atypical genital nevi. J Cutan Pathol 2008;35(Suppl. 2):24–7.

[42] Ferrari A, Zalaudek I, Argenziano G, Buccini P, De Simone P, Silipo V, et al. Dermoscopy of pigmented lesions of the vulva: a retrospective morphological study. Dermatology 2011;222:157–66.

[43] Bravo Puccio F, Chian C. Acral junctional nevus versus acral lentiginous melanoma in situ: a differential diagnosis that should be based on clinicopathologic correlation. Arch Pathol Lab Med 2011;135:847–52.

[44] LeBoit PE. A diagnosis for maniacs. Am J Dermatopathol 2000;22:556–8.

[45] Fabrizi G, Pagliarello C, Parente P, Massi G. Atypical nevi of the scalp in adolescents. J Cutan Pathol 2007;34:365–9.

[46] Schaffer JV, Glusac EJ, Bolognia JL. The eclipse naevus: tan centre with stellate brown rim. Br J Dermatol 2001;145:1023–6.

[47] Khalifeh I, Taraif S, Reed JA, Lazar AF, Diwan AH, Prieto VG. A subgroup of melanocytic nevi on the distal lower extremity (ankle) shares features of acral nevi, dysplastic nevi, and melanoma in situ: a potential misdiagnosis of melanoma in situ. Am J Surg Pathol 2007;31:1130–6.

[48] Rongioletti F, Ball RA, Marcus R, Barnhill RL. Histopathological features of flexural melanocytic nevi: a study of 40 cases. J Cutan Pathol 2000;27:215–7.

[49] Rongioletti F, Urso C, Batolo D, Chimenti S, Fanti PA, Filotico R, et al. Melanocytic nevi of the breast: a histologic case–control study. J Cutan Pathol 2004;31:137–40.

[50] Saad AG, Patel S, Mutasim DF. Melanocytic nevi of the auricular region: histologic characteristics and diagnostic difficulties. Am J Dermatopathol 2005;27:111–5.

[51] Lazova R, Lester B, Glusac EJ, Handerson T, McNiff J. The characteristic histopathologic features of nevi on and around the ear. J Cutan Pathol 2005;32:40–4.

[52] Zembowicz A, Mandal RV, Choopong P. Melanocytic lesions of the conjunctiva. Arch Pathol Lab Med 2010;134:1785–92.

[53] Elder DE, Xu X. The approach to the patient with a difficult melanocytic lesion. Pathology 2004;36:428–34.

[54] Smith KJ, Barrett TL, Skelton HG 3rd, Lupton GP, Graham JH. Spindle cell and epithelioid cell nevi with atypia and metastasis (malignant Spitz nevus). Am J Surg Pathol 1989;13:931–9.

[55] Zembowicz A, Scolyer RA. Nevus/melanocytoma/melanoma: an emerging paradigm for classification of melanocytic neoplasms? Arch Pathol Lab Med 2011;135:300–6.

[56] Magro CM, Abraham RM, Guo R, Li S, Wang X, Proper S, et al. Deep penetrating nevus-like borderline tumors: a unique subset of ambiguous melanocytic tumors with malignant potential and normal cytogenetics. Eur J Dermatol 2014;24:594–602.

[57] Luo S, Sepehr A, Tsao H. Spitz nevi and other spitzoid lesions part II: natural history and management. J Am Acad Dermatol 2011;65:1087–92.

[58] Lallas A, Krygidis A, Ferrara G, Kittler H, Apalla Z, Castagnetti F, et al. Atypical Spitz tumours and sentinel lymph node biopsy: a systematic review. Lancet Oncol 2014;15:e178–83.

[59] Da Forno PD, Prngle JH, Fletcher A, Bamford M, Su L, Potter L, et al. BRAF, NRAS and HRAS mutations in spitzoid tumors and their pathogenetic significance. Br J Dermatol 2009;161:364–72.

[60] Blokx W, van Dijk MC, Ruiter DJ. Molecular cytogenetics of cutaneous melanocytic lesions: diagnostic, prognostic and therapeutic aspects. Histopathology 2010;56: 121–32.

[61] Whiteman DC, Pavan WJ, Bastian BC. The melanomas: a synthesis of epidemiological, clinical, histopathological, genetic, and biological aspects, supporting distinct subtypes, causal pathways, and cells of origin. Pigment Cell Melanoma Res 2011;24:879–97.

[62] van Engen-van Grunsven AC, Kusters-Vandevelde H, Groenen PJ, Blokx WA. Update on molecular pathology of cutaneous melanocytic lesions: what is new in diagnosis and molecular testing for treatment? Front Med (Lausanne) 2014;1:39.

[63] Zembowicz A, Carney JA, Mihm MC. Pigmented epithelioid melanocytoma: a low-grade melanocytic tumor with metastatic potential indistinguishable from animal-type melanoma and epithelioid blue nevus. Am J Surg Pathol 2004;28:31–40.

[64] Carney JA, Ferreiro JA. The epithelioid blue nevus. A multicentric familial tumor with important associations, including cardiac myxoma and psammomatous melanotic schwannoma. Am J Surg Pathol 1996;20:259–72.

[65] Kirschner LS, Sandrini F, Monbo J, Lin JP, Carney JA, Stratakis CA. Genetic heterogeneity and spectrum of mutations of the PRKAR1A gene in patients with the Carney complex. Hum Mol Gen 2000;9:3037–46.

[66] McFadyean J. Equine melanosis. J Comp Pathol Ther 1933;46:186–2004.

[67] Ludgate MW, Fullen DR, Lee J, Rees R, Sabe MS, Wong SL, et al. Animal-type melanoma: a clinical and histopathological study of 22 cases from a single institution. Br J Dermatol 2010;162:129–36.

[68] Moscarella E, Ricci R, Argenziano G, Lallas A, Longo C, Lombardi M, et al. Pigmented epithelioid melanocytoma: clinical, dermoscopic, and histopathologic features. Br J Dermatol 2016;174:1115–7.

[69] Seab JA Jr, Graham JH, Helwig EB. Deep penetrating nevus. Am J Surg Pathol 1989;13:39–44.

[70] Cooper PH. Deep penetrating (plexiform spindle cell) nevus. A frequent participant in combined nevus. J Cutan Pathol 1992;19:172–80.

[71] Robson A, Morley-Quante M, Hempel H, McKee PH, Calonje E. Deep penetrating naevus: clinicopathological study of 31 cases with further delineation of histological features allowing distinction from other pigmented benign melanocytic lesions and melanoma. Histopathology 2003;43:529–37.

[72] Prieto VG, Shea CR. Immunohistochemistry of melanocytic proliferations. Arch Pathol Lab Med 2011;135:853–9.

[73] Braun-Falco M, Schempp W, Weyers W. Molecular diagnosis in dermatopathology: what makes sense, and what doesn't. Exp Dermatol 2009;18:12–23.

[74] Dadras SS. Molecular diagnostics in melanoma: current status and perspectives. Arch Pathol Lab Med 2011;135:860–9.

[75] Pinkel D, Segraves R, Sudar D, Clark S, Poole I, Kowbel D, et al. High resolution analysis of DNA copy number variation using comparative genomic hybridization to microarrays. Nat Genet 1998;20:207–11.

[76] Bastian BC, LeBoit PE, Hamm H, Brocker EB, Pinkel D. Chromosomal gains and losses in primary cutaneous melanomas detected by comparative genomic hybridization. Cancer Res 1998;58:2170–5.

[77] Bastian BC, Wesselmann U, Pinkel D, LeBoit PE. Molecular cytogenetic analysis of Spitz nevi shows clear differences to melanoma. J Invest Dermatol 1999;113:1065–9.

[78] Bastian BC, Olshen AB, LeBoit PE, Pinkel D. Classifying melanocytic tumors based on DNA copy number changes. Am J Pathol 2003;163:1765–70.

[79] Bastian BC, LeBoit PE, Pinkel D. Mutations and copy number increase of HRAS in Spitz nevi with distinctive histopathological features. Am J Pathol 2000;157:967–72.

[80] Harvell JD, Kohler S, Zhu S, Hernandez-Boussard T, Pollack JR, van de Rijn M. High-resolution array-based comparative genomic hybridization for distinguishing paraffin-embedded Spitz nevi and melanomas. Diagn Mol Pathol 2004;13:22–5.

[81] Bauer J, Bastian BC. Distinguishing melanocytic nevi from melanoma by DNA copy number changes: comparative genomic hybridization as a research and diagnostic tool. Dermatol Ther 2006;19:40–9.

[82] Ali L, Helm T, Cheney R, Conroy J, Sait S, Guitart J, et al. Correlating array comparative genomic hybridization findings with histology and outcome in spitzoid melanocytic neoplasms. Int J Clin Exp Pathol 2010;3:593–9.

[83] Krauthammer M, Kong Y, Bacchiocchi A, Evans P, Pornputtapong N, Wu C, et al. Exome sequencing identifies recurrent mutations in NF1 and RASopathy genes in sun-exposed melanomas. Nat Genet 2015;47:996–1002.

[84] Lee S, Barnhill RL, Dummer R, Dalton J, Wu J, Pappo A, et al. TERT promoter mutations are predictive of aggressive clinical behavior in patients with spitzoid melanocytic neoplasms. Sci Rep 2015;5:11200.

[85] Gerami P, Jewell SS, Morrison LE, Blondin B, Schulz J, Ruffalo T, et al. Fluorescence in situ hybridization (FISH) as an ancillary diagnostic tool in the diagnosis of melanoma. Am J Surg Pathol 2009;33:1146–56.

[86] Gerami P, Mafee M, Lurtsbarapa T, Guitart J, Haghighat Z, Newman M. Sensitivity of fluorescence in situ hybridization for melanoma diagnosis using RREB1, MYB, Cep6, and 11q13 probes in melanoma subtypes. Arch Dermatol 2010;146:273–8.

[87] Ferrara G, De Vanna AC. Fluorescence in-situ hybridization for melanoma diagnosis: a review and a reappraisal. Am J Dermatopathol 2016;38:253–69.

[88] Gerami P, Li G, Pouryazdanparast P, Blondin B, Beilfuss B, Slenk C, et al. A highly specific and discriminatory FISH assay for distinguishing between benign and malignant melanocytic neoplasms. Am J Surg Pathol 2012;36:808–17.

[89] Gerami P, Scolyer RA, Xu X, Elder DE, Abraham RM, Fullen D, et al. Risk assessment of atypical spitzoid melanocytic neoplasms using FISH to identify chromosomal copy number aberrations. Am J Surg Pathol 2013;37:676–84.

[90] Wiesner T, He J, Yelensky R, Esteve-Puig R, Botton T, Yeh I, et al. Kinase fusions are frequent in Spitz tumours and spitzoid melanomas. Nat Comm 2014;5:3116.

[91] Ferrara G, Argenyi Z, Argenziano G, Cerio R, Cerroni L, Di Blasi A, et al. The influence of the clinical information in the histopathologic diagnosis of melanocytic skin neoplasms. PLoS One 2009;4:e5375.

[92] Ferrara G, Annessi G, Argenyi Z, Argenziano G, Beltraminelli H, Cerio R, et al. Prior knowledge of the clinical picture does not introduce bias in the histopathologic diagnosis of melanocytic skin lesions. J Cutan Pathol 2015;. [Epub ahead of print].

[93] Haspeslagh M, Degryse N, De Wispelaere I. Routine use of ex vivo dermoscopy with "derm dotting" in dermatopathology. Am J Dermatopathol 2013;35:867–9.

[94] Longo C, Piana S, Lallas A, Moscarella E, Lombardi M, Raucci M, et al. Routine clinical–pathological correlation of pigmented skin tumors can influence patient management. PLoS One 2015;10:e0136031.

[95] Pathology reports, <http://www.cancer.gov/about-cancer/diagnosis-staging/diagnosis/pathology-reports-fact-sheet> [accessed Dec 31, 2015].

[96] Ferrara G, Misciali C, Brenn T, Cerroni L, Kazakov DW, Perasole A, et al. The impact of molecular morphology techniques on the expert diagnosis in melanocytic skin neoplasms. Int J Surgical Pathol 2013;21:483–92.

[97] Ferrara G, Argenziano G, Soyer HP, Corona R, Sera F, Brunetti B, et al. Dermoscopic and histopathologic diagnosis of equivocal melanocytic skin lesions. An interdisciplinary study on 107 cases. Cancer 2002;95:1094–100.

[98] LeBoit PE. What do these cells prove? Am J Dermatopathol 2003;25:355–6.
[99] Ferrara G, Errico ME, Donofrio V, Zalaudek I, Argenziano G. Melanocytic tumors of uncertain malignant potential in childhood: do we really need sentinel node biopsy? J Cutan Pathol 2012;39:1049–51.
[100] Jones EL, Jones TS, Pearlman NW, Gao D, Stovall R, Gajdos C, et al. Long-term follow-up and survival of patients following a recurrence of melanoma after a negative sentinel node biopsy result. JAMA Surg 2013;16:1–6.
[101] Smith LB. Pathology review of outside material: when does it help and when can it hurt? J Clin Oncol 2011;29:2724–7.

Further Reading

Bender RP, McGinniss MJ, Esmay P, Velazquez EF. Identification of HRAS mutations and absence of GNAQ or GNA11 mutations in deep penetrating nevi. Mod Pathol 2013;26:1320–8.

Murali R, Wiesner T, Rosenblum MK, Bastian BC. GNAQ and GNA11 mutations in melanocytomas of the central nervous system. Acta Neuropathol 2012;123:457–9.

Indsto JO, Kumar S, Wang L, Crotty KA, Arbuckle SM, Mann GJ. Low prevalence of RAS-RAF mutations in Spitz melanocytic nevi compared with other melanocytic lesions. J Cutan Pathol 2007;34:448–55.

Van Raamsdonk CD, Griewank KG, Crosby MB, Garrido MC, Vemula S, Wiesner T, et al. Mutations in GNA11 in uveal melanoma. N Engl J Med 2010;363:2191–9.

Zembowicz A, Phadke PA. Blue nevi and variants: an update. Arch Pathol Lab Med 2011;135:327–36.

S U B C H A P T E R

7.2

Familial Melanoma and Multiple Primary Melanoma

Maria Concetta Fargnoli*, Cristina Pellegrini*, Ketty Peris**

*University of L'Aquila, L'Aquila, Italy
**Institute of Dermatology, Catholic University of the Sacred Heart, Rome, Italy

Hereditary melanoma predisposition is suggested by:

1. Families with more than one member with melanoma
2. Occurrence of multiple primary melanomas (MPMs) in one individual

1. Familial melanoma is defined as follows:
   a. A family in which two first-degree relatives are diagnosed with melanoma
   b. Families with three or more melanoma patients on the same side of the family (irrespective of degree of relationship):
   c. In these families the pattern of susceptibility is consistent with an autosomal dominant inheritance with incomplete penetrance.
   d. An estimated 5%–10% of all cutaneous melanoma cases occur in families.
2. MPMs:
   a. Approximately 3.5%–5.5% of all patients with melanoma will develop additional primary melanomas in their lifetime [1–5].
   b. Patients with melanoma have approximately a ninefold risk of developing a subsequent melanoma compared with the general population [2], with the highest risk for patients who had their first melanoma before the age of 40 years [6].
   c. The risk of subsequent primary melanomas decreases with increasing latency but remains quite elevated more than 20 years after diagnosis of a first primary melanoma, supporting continued long-term surveillance in melanoma survivors with complete skin examination [2].

1 MELANOMA SUSCEPTIBILITY GENES AND CLINICAL PREDICTORS OF GERMLINE MUTATIONS

Genes that predispose to melanoma are typically grouped in high-, medium-, and low-penetrance genes. Penetrance relates to the lifetime risk of developing melanoma for a mutation carrier and reflects the overall contribution of a specific gene alteration to melanoma risk.

Susceptibility for approximately 50% of melanoma families is due to mutations in one of the following high-penetrance melanoma predisposition genes (Table 7.2.1) [7,8]:

- *CDKN2A* [7–10]:
  - This gene encodes two different proteins in alternative reading frames:
    - The α transcript encoding the p16^{INK4A} protein, which regulates the G1-phase exit by inhibiting the CDK4-mediated phosphorylation of the retinoblastoma protein
    - The β transcript encoding the alternative protein p14^{ARF}, which acts via the p53 pathway to induce cell cycle arrest or apoptosis:
      - Both p53 and p16 have roles in responses to UV damage and cellular senescence.
  - Twenty to 40% of melanoma families have germinal *CDKN2A* mutations [11–17].

TABLE 7.2.1 High- and Medium-Penetrance Melanoma Susceptibility Genes, Contribution to Melanoma Predisposition and Associated Cancers

Gene penetrance	Gene	Encoded protein and role	Year	Mutation prevalence [7]		Associated cancers	References
High penetrance	Cyclin-dependent kinase inhibitor 2A (CDKN2A)	Two unrelated proteins from alternatively spliced transcripts (p16^{INK4A} and p14^{ARF}), both involved in cell cycle regulation	1994	P16^{INK4A}	≈20%–40% of families	Pancreatic carcinoma	[9,10,12,13]
				P14^{ARF}	≈1% of families	Neural system tumors	[30,31]
	Cyclin-dependent kinase 4 (CDK4)	A protein kinase involved in cell cycle G1-S phase transition	1996	17 families		—	[20,21]
	BRCA1-associated protein-1 (BAP1)	A deubiquitinating enzyme that acts as transcriptional repressor for silencing of genes regulating cell fate determination and stem cell pluripotency	2010	24 families		Uveal melanoma, mesothelioma, renal cell carcinoma, basal cell carcinoma	[22-25]
	Telomerase reverse-transcriptase (TERT)	The catalytic subunit of the telomerase complex that prevents the progressive shortening of the telomeres	2013	1 family		—	[26]

(Continued)

TABLE 7.2.1　High- and Medium-Penetrance Melanoma Susceptibility Genes, Contribution to Melanoma Predisposition and Associated Cancers (cont.)

Gene penetrance	Gene	Encoded protein and role	Year	Mutation prevalence [7]	Associated cancers	References
	Protection of telomeres 1 (POT1)	Members of the six-component protein complex of the shelterin, which protects telomeres from being mistakenly recognized as DNA breaks, regulating telomere region DNA replication and telomerase recruitment and activity	2014	12 families	Glioma	[27,28]
	Adrenocortical dysplasia homologue (ACD)		2014	6 families	—	[29]
	Telomeric repeat binding factor 2 (TERF2IP)		2014	5 families	—	[29]
Intermediate penetrance	Melanocortin 1 receptor (MC1R)	A transmembrane-G protein–coupled receptor that binds to α-MSH involved in eumelanin pigment synthesis and melanocyte proliferation	2001	na	—	[32,33]
	Microphthalmia-associated transcription factor (MITF)	A transcription factor that regulates differentiation and development of melanocytes	2011	na	Renal cell carcinoma	[34,35]

na, Not applicable.

TABLE 7.2.2   Clinical Predictors That Help Identifying Appropriate Candidates for Genetic Evaluation

Clinical feature	
Family history of melanoma	If two or three cases of melanoma within a family depending on the incidence of melanoma in the specific population
Multiple primary melanoma	The likelihood of detecting a mutation increases with the increasing number of primaries in an individual
Pancreatic cancer	Diagnosis of pancreatic cancer in a melanoma family
Early age at melanoma onset	No genetic testing indicated as isolated feature

- The penetrance in *CDKN2A* mutation carriers is very high, ranging from 58% in Europe to 76% in the United States and to 91% in Australia by age 80 years [18].
- Detection of a *CDKN2A* mutation in melanoma families increases with [13]:
  - The number of affected members (approximately 10% for two-case melanoma families and 30%–40% for families with three or more cases of melanoma)
  - The presence of relatives with multiple primaries, pancreatic cancer
  - Early age at onset (Table 7.2.2; Fig. 7.2.1)
- Among MPM patients, the prevalence of *CDKN2A* mutations is higher in the presence of family history than in sporadic MPM patients and increases with the number of primary melanomas diagnosed in the individual [14,17].
- Younger age at melanoma onset is a weak predictor of *CDKN2A* mutations in a nonfamilial setting [19].
- *CDK4*:
  - This gene encodes one of the binding partners of p16 [20].
  - The phenotype of *CDK4*-mutated families is indistinguishable from the *CDKN2A* phenotype [21].
- *BAP1*:
  - The *BAP1* gene is a critical regulator of oncogenesis.
  - *BAP1* cancer susceptibility syndrome [22–25]:
    - Multiple skin-colored spitzoid melanocytic tumors
    - Uveal melanoma
    - Cutaneous melanoma
    - Mesothelioma
    - Renal cell carcinoma
    - Basal cell carcinoma

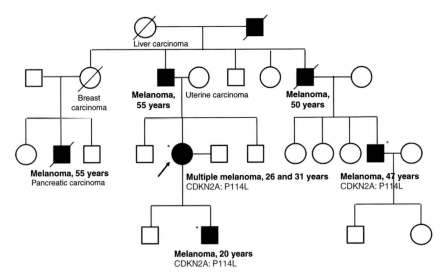

FIGURE 7.2.1   **Pedigree of a *CDKN2A*-mutated family with seven affected members.**
The pedigree should span three generations and note both maternal and paternal relatives
either affected or unaffected with melanoma or other cancers including type of cancer and
age of diagnosis.

- *TERT* gene mutation, encoding the catalytic subunit of telomerase, has been identified in one family [26].
- *POT1*, *ACD*, and *TERF2IP* mutations account for approximately 9% of high-density families lacking mutations in known high-penetrance genes [27–29].

The underlying genetic basis is unexplained for the remaining half of highly dense melanoma families:

- In these cases a polygenic susceptibility as a result of coinheritance of multiple medium- and/or low-risk alleles or interplay between susceptibility genes and genetic modifiers (other genes, phenotypic characteristics, and environmental risk factors) has been suggested.
- To date two medium-penetrance genes (*MC1R* and *MITF*) predisposing to melanoma have been identified (Table 7.2.1):
  - *MC1R* gene encodes the melanocyte-stimulating hormone receptor.
    - It has a key role in cutaneous pigmentation [36].
    - *MC1R* variants, mainly RHC alleles, have been shown to contribute to melanoma development independently of phenotypic features [32].
    - Notably, a stronger MC1R/melanoma association has been reported for patients with darkly pigmented skin, supporting a nonpigment pathway for MC1R to cause melanoma [32].

- Coinheritance of *MC1R* variants with *CDKN2A* mutations increases the penetrance of melanoma in *CDKN2A* mutation-positive families [33].
- The *MITF* gene is a master regulator gene of melanocyte development and differentiation and has been associated with melanoma development and progression [37].
  - The recurrent germline E318K mutation of the *MITF* gene has been implicated in familial melanoma and in melanoma/renal cell carcinoma susceptibility. This mutation has been linked to a particular phenotype characterized by nonblue eye color, increased number of nevi, and MPM [34–35].

2 MELANOMA SUSCEPTIBILITY GENES AND ASSOCIATED CANCERS

Some melanoma susceptibility genes have been linked to risk of other cancers (Table 7.2.1):

- *CDKN2A* and pancreatic cancer [12]:
  - Patients should be aware of the current lack of effective screening guidelines.
- *CDKN2A* and other tobacco-associated cancers (respiratory and upper digestive cancers) [17–29,32–35,37,38]:
  - Patients should avoid smoking.
- *BAP1* cancer susceptibility syndrome [22–25]:
- *MITF* and renal cell carcinoma [34,35]
- *POT1* and glioma [39]

3 GENETIC TESTING AND COUNSELING

Genetic counseling can be offered to melanoma patients with hereditary predisposition to better understand [40,41]:

- The meaning of the disease
- The pattern of inheritance
- The option of genetic testing
- The possible results and implications for other family members
- Recommendation for primary and secondary prevention of melanoma
- Psychological assessment

To select appropriate candidates eligible for genetic testing in melanoma with regard to the specific population (Table 7.2.3):

- The rule of two for countries with low incidence of melanoma (southern Europe) may be suggested [19].

TABLE 7.2.3 Selection Criteria for Genetic Testing According to Melanoma
Incidence [19]

Area/population with low melanoma incidence:

• Two (synchronous or metachronous) primary melanomas in an individual and/or
• Families with the following clinical features in first- or second-degree relatives on the
same side of the family:
  ◦ Two cases of melanoma (one invasive) or
  ◦ One case of melanoma and one case of pancreatic cancer

Area/population with moderate- to high-melanoma incidence:

• Three primary melanomas in an individual and/or
• Families with the following clinical features in first- or second-degree relatives on the
same side of the family:
  ◦ Three cases of melanoma (one invasive) or
  ◦ Two cases of melanoma and one case of pancreatic cancer or
  ◦ One case of melanoma and two cases of pancreatic cancer

• The rule of three for countries with moderate–high incidence of
  melanoma (the United States and northern Europe) may be suggested.
• A rule of four for countries with very high incidence of melanoma
  (Australia) may be suggested [40].

If a mutation in a melanoma susceptibility gene is detected in a family,
screening of other members of the family is recommended.

If no *CDKN2A* mutation is identified within a melanoma family, it
should be stressed that the family is still at increased risk of melanoma on
the basis of the family history.

In the future, if clinical utility of genetic testing will be demonstrated,
high-penetrance predisposition genes might be included in gene panels
for melanoma risk evaluation. Routine screening of medium- or low-penetrance gene is less likely due to uncertainty of predicting clinical outcome
of disease development.

References

[1] McCaul KA, Fritschi L, Baade P, Coory M. The incidence of second primary invasive
melanoma in Queensland, 1982–2003. Cancer Causes Control 2008;19:451–8.

[2] Bradford PT, Freedman DM, Goldstein AM, Tucker MA. Increased risk of second primary cancers after a diagnosis of melanoma. Arch Dermatol 2010;146:265–72.

[3] Chen T, Fallah M, Försti A, Kharazmi E, Sundquist K, Hemminki K. Risk of next melanoma in patients with familial and sporadic melanoma by number of previous melanomas. JAMA Dermatol 2015;151:607–15.

[4] Chen T, Hemminki K, Kharazmi E, Ji J, Sundquist K, Fallah M. Multiple primary (even
in situ) melanomas in a patient pose significant risk to family members. Eur J Cancer
2014;50:2659–67.

[5] Ferrone CR, Ben Porat L, Panageas KS, et al. Clinicopathological features of and risk
factors for multiple primary melanomas. JAMA 2005;294:1647–54.

[6] van der Rhee JI, Krijnen P, Gruis NA, et al. Clinical and histologic characteristics of malignant melanoma in families with a germline mutation in CDKN2A. J Am Acad Dermatol 2011;65:281–8.

[7] Aoude LG, Wadt KA, Pritchard AL, Hayward NK. Genetics of familial melanoma: 20 years after CDKN2A. Pigment Cell Melanoma Res 2015;28:148–60.

[8] Read J, Wadt KA, Hayward NK. Melanoma genetics. J Med Genet 2016;53:1–14.

[9] Hussussian CJ, Struewing JP, Goldstein AM, et al. Germline p16 mutations in familial melanoma. Nat Genet 1994;8:15–21.

[10] Kamb A, Shattuck-Eidens D, Eeles R, et al. Analysis of the p16 gene (CDKN2) as a candidate for the chromosome 9p melanoma susceptibility locus. Nat Genet 1994;8: 23–6.

[11] Begg CB, Orlow I, Hummer AJ, et al. Lifetime risk of melanoma in CDKN2A mutation carriers in a population-based sample. J Natl Cancer Inst 2005;97:1507–15.

[12] Goldstein AM, Chan M, Harland M, et al. High-risk melanoma susceptibility genes and pancreatic cancer, neural system tumors, and uveal melanoma across GenoMEL. Cancer Res 2006;66:9818–28.

[13] Goldstein AM, Chan M, Harland M, et al. Features associated with germline CDKN2A mutations: a GenoMEL study of melanoma-prone families from three continents. J Med Genet 2007;44:99–106.

[14] Bruno W, Ghiorzo P, Battistuzzi L, et al. Clinical genetic testing for familial melanoma in Italy: a cooperative study. J Am Acad Dermatol 2009;61:775–82.

[15] Maubec E, Chaudru V, Mohamdi H, et al. Familial melanoma: clinical factors associated with germline CDKN2A mutations according to the number of patients affected by melanoma in a family. J Am Acad Dermatol 2012;67:1257–64.

[16] Harland M, Cust AE, Badenas C, et al. Prevalence and predictors of germline CDKN2A mutations for melanoma cases from Australia, Spain and the United Kingdom. Hered Cancer Clin Pract 2014;12:20.

[17] Potrony M, Puig-Butillé JA, Aguilera P, et al. Increased prevalence of lung, breast, and pancreatic cancers in addition to melanoma risk in families bearing the cyclin-dependent kinase inhibitor 2A mutation: implications for genetic counseling. J Am Acad Dermatol 2014;71:888–95.

[18] Bishop DT, Demenais F, Goldstein AM, et al. Geographical variation in the penetrance of CDKN2A mutations for melanoma. J Natl Cancer Inst 2002;94:894–903.

[19] Leachman SA, Carucci J, Kohlmann W, et al. Selection criteria for genetic assessment of patients with familial melanoma. J Am Acad Dermatol 2009;61:677.e1–677.e14.

[20] Zuo L, Weger J, Yang Q, et al. Germline mutations in the p16INK4a binding domain of CDK4 in familial melanoma. Nat. Genet 1996;12:97–9.

[21] Puntervoll HE, Yang XR, Vetti HH, et al. Melanoma prone families with CDK4 germline mutation: phenotypic profile and associations with MC1R variants. J Med Genet. 2013;50:264–70.

[22] Wiesner T, Obenauf AC, Murali R, et al. Germline mutations in BAP1 predispose to melanocytic tumors. Nat Genet 2011;43:1018–21.

[23] Testa JR, Cheung M, Pei J, et al. Germline BAP1 mutations predispose to malignant mesothelioma. Nat Genet 2011;43:1022–5.

[24] Popova T, Hebert L, Jacquemin V, et al. Germline BAP1 mutations predispose to renal cell carcinomas. Am J Hum Genet 2013;92:974–80.

[25] Wadt KA, Aoude LG, Johansson P, et al. A recurrent germline BAP1 mutation and extension of the BAP1 tumor predisposition spectrum to include basal cell carcinoma. Clin Genet 2015;88:267–72.

[26] Horn S, Figl A, Rachakonda PS, Fischer C, et al. TERT promoter mutations in familial and sporadic melanoma. Science 2013;339:959–61.

[27] Shi J, Yang XR, Ballew B, et al. Rare missense variants in POT1 predispose to familial cutaneous malignant melanoma. Nat Genet 2014;46:482–6.

[28] Robles-Espinoza CD, Harland M, Ramsay AJ, et al. POT1 loss-of-function variants predispose to familial melanoma. Nat Genet 2014;46:478–81.

[29] Aoude LG, Pritchard AL, Robles-Espinoza CD, et al. Nonsense mutations in the shelterin complex genes ACD and TERF2IP in familial melanoma. J Natl Cancer Inst 2014;13(2):107.

[30] Azizi E, Friedman J, Pavlotsky F, Iscovich J, et al. Familial cutaneous malignant melanoma and tumors of the nervous system. A hereditary cancer syndrome. Cancer 1995;76:1571–8.

[31] Bahuau M, Vidaud D, Jenkins RB, et al. Germ-line deletion involving the INK4 locus in familial proneness to melanoma and nervous system tumors. Cancer Res 1998;58:2298–303.

[32] Pasquali E, García-Borrón JC, Fargnoli MC, et al. MC1R variants increased the risk of sporadic cutaneous melanoma in darker-pigmented Caucasians: a pooled-analysis from the M-SKIP project. Int J Cancer 2015;136:618–31.

[33] Fargnoli MC, Gandini S, Peris K, Maisonneuve P, Raimondi S. MC1R variants increase melanoma risk in families with CDKN2A mutations: a meta-analysis. Eur J Cancer 2010;46:1413–20.

[34] Bertolotto C, Lesueur F, Giuliano S, et al. A SUMOylation-defective MITF germline mutation predisposes to melanoma and renal carcinoma. Nature 2011;480:94–8.

[35] Yokoyama S, Woods SL, Boyle GM, et al. A novel recurrent mutation in MITF predisposes to familial and sporadic melanoma. Nature 2011;480:99–103.

[36] Beaumont KA, Shekar SN, Newton RA, et al. Receptor function, dominant negative activity and phenotype correlations for MC1R variant alleles. Hum Mol Genet 2007;16:2249–60.

[37] Levy C, Khaled M, Fisher DE. MITF: master regulator of melanocyte development and melanoma oncogene. Trends Mol Med 2006;12:406–14.

[38] Helgadottir H, Höiom V, Jönsson G, et al. High risk of tobacco-related cancers in CDKN2A mutation-positive melanoma families. J Med Genet 2014;51:545–52.

[39] Bainbridge MN, Armstrong GN, Gramatges MM, et al. Germline mutations in shelterin complex genes are associated with familial glioma. J Natl Cancer Ins 2014;107:384.

[40] Badenas C, Aguilera P, Puig-Butillé JA, Carrera C, Malvehy J, Puig S. Genetic counseling in melanoma. Dermatol Ther 2012;25:397–402.

[41] Gabree M, Patel D, Rodgers L. Clinical applications of melanoma genetics. Curr Treat Options Oncol 2014;15:336–50.

SUBCHAPTER

7.3

Pregnancy and Melanoma

Athanassios Kyrgidis, *Aimilios Lallas*

Aristotle University of Thessaloniki, Thessaloniki, Greece

1 EPIDEMIOLOGY OF PREGNANCY-ASSOCIATED MELANOMA (PAM)

- Melanoma is the most common malignancy encountered during pregnancy, accounting for 31% of all malignancies diagnosed in pregnant women [1].
- In Australia, the crude incidence of PAM increased from 37.1 per 100,000 maternities in 1994 to 51.8 per 100,000 maternities in 2008 [2].
- No association between women's parity and melanoma has been reported [3].
- Case reports with unfavorable prognosis have been published and still emerge [4–6]. However, to-date reviews have not been able to conclude whether pregnancy influences the prognosis of melanoma [7–10]. Within the past couple of years, two large epidemiological cohort studies have been published. The first, from the United Kingdom, reported on a significantly increased risk [3], while the second one, from Sweden, was not able to document such a correlation [11].

In this chapter, using evidence gathered for a synchronous review by some of the authors of this book [12], we present a systematic effort to gather all available evidence and attempt a metaanalysis of this existing evidence with regard to the prognosis of melanoma diagnosed during pregnancy or postpartum, as compared with melanoma in female patients not related to pregnancy.

The prespecified outcomes of this most recent systematic review were as follows: primary outcome was overall survival (OS) of female patients pregnant or not when diagnosed with melanoma, disease-specific survival (DSS), disease-free survival (DFS), and time to recurrence.

The statistical methods used in the latter review [12] were those reported in the Cochrane Handbook, using Review Manager 5 software [Review Manager (RevMan), Oxford, England: The Cochrane Collaboration, 2011].

This work, using appropriate metaanalysis methodology, presented for the first time robust evidence that melanoma diagnosed during pregnancy is associated with increased mortality [12]. Because of the statistical approach, this metaanalysis integrated data from all available studies, including those not reporting hazard ratios (HRs), minimizing, therefore, selection bias due to convenient sampling.

2 MAIN RESULTS

- Overall, 17 relevant studies were finally included in the qualitative synthesis (Table 7.3.1). Calculation of HRs was possible for 15 studies, which were eligible for the quantitative syntheses. Of the 15 eligible studies, 13 reported on OS [3,13–24] and 2 studies reported on DSS [11,25]. Among the 15 included studies, 4 reported on both OS and DFS [13,15,19,20]. These studies were included in both quantitative syntheses for OS and DFS.
- Among the nine case–control studies [13,15–17,19,20,22,23], two did not include matching of cases to controls [15,19], two included age matching [13,17], and four [20,22–24] included stage and/or tumor thickness matching. McManamny et al. reported no matching but post hoc comparison for melanoma thickness, which was not significant between cases and controls [16]. Among the six cohort studies [3,11,14,18,21,25], Stensheim et al. reported HRs also after adjustment for tumor stage and age [25]; Moller et al. reported HRs also after adjustment for tumor stage [3] while Johansson et al. reported HRs also after adjustment for age [11].

2.1 Outcomes

- Most studies (and mainly the older ones) do not report HRs between groups in comparison. Instead, they provide survival proportions at specified intervals, median survival, or log-rank P values. All studies include crude survival Kaplan–Meier curves for groups of interest.
- Fig. 7.3.1 presents the included studies, and corresponding HRs and 95% CIs for OS. We found that PAM is associated with a 17% higher mortality as compared to melanoma diagnosed in female patients not associated with pregnancy (total HR = 1.17, 95% CI: 1.03–1.33, P = .02).
- Fig. 7.3.2 presents included studies, and corresponding HRs and 95% CIs for DFS. We found that PAM is associated with a 50% higher recurrence rate, as compared to melanoma diagnosed in female patients not associated with pregnancy (total HR = 1.50, 95% CI: 1.19–1.90, P < .001). The heterogeneity associated with this test was low (P = .69; I^2 = 0%).

TABLE 7.3.1 Summary of the 17 Studies Included in the Systematic Review

No.	Study	Year	Place	Design	Outcome	Total number of patients in the study	Melanoma diagnosis in relation to pregnancy (PAM definition in each study)	Number of PAM cases	Number of MM controls	Stage	Matching	Breslow's thickness, PAM (mm)	Breslow's thickness, MM (mm)	Mean age, PAM (years)	Mean age, MM (years)	Mean*, follow-up time (years)	NOS scoring
1	Reintgen et al.	1985	Duke University Comprehensive Cancer Center, Durham, NC	Case–control	OS, DSS	1,026	During pregnancy	58	585	1	None	1.9	1.51	29.2	33.1	5	5
2	McManamny et al.	1989	Frenchay Hospital, Bristol	Case–control	OS	264	During pregnancy	23	241	1	None, post hoc not significant for thickness	1.62 (survived), 2.62 (died)	1.72 (survived), 3.96 (died)	28.7	32.3	2 months to 20 years	6
3	Wong et al.	1989	John Wayne Cancer Clinic, UCLA	Case–control	OS	685	During pregnancy	66	619	1	Computer aided: age, tumor depth, anatomic, histopathological	1.24	128	28	31		6
4	Slingluff et al.	1990	Duke University Comprehensive Cancer Center, Durham, NC	Case–control	OS, DSS	186	During pregnancy	100	86	1, 2, 3	Age, stage, anatomic, histology, tumor depth, Clark's level, ulceration	2.17	1.52	28.9	29.6	6	6

(Continued)

TABLE 7.3.1 Summary of the 17 Studies Included in the Systematic Review (cont.)

No.	Study	Year	Place	Design	Outcome	Total number of patients in the study	Melanoma diagnosis in relation to pregnancy (PAM definition in each study)	Number of PAM cases	Number of MM controls	Stage	Matching	Breslow's thickness, PAM (mm)	Breslow's thickness, MM (mm)	Mean age, PAM (years)	Mean age, MM (years)	Mean*, follow-up time (years)	NOS scoring
5	MacKie et al.	1991	University of Glasgow, Istituto Tumori di Milano, Tulane University	Case–control	OS, DSS	388	During pregnancy but versus (1) before, (2) after, (3) between	92	296	1		2.38	1.71				5
6	Lens et al.	2004	Swedish National Cancer and Mortality Registry	Cohort	OS	5,535	During pregnancy	185	5,348		Breslow's thickness, Clark's level, and tumor site	1.28	1.07	29.3	35	11.6 years (median)	6
7	O'Meara et al.	2005	California Office of State-Wide Health Planning and Development, SEER	Cohort	OS	2,863	During pregnancy or within the first year postpartum	412	2,451	All	Age	0.855	0.81			10 years (maximum)	6
8	Miller et al.	2010	Tel-Aviv Sourasky Medical Center	Case–control	OS	76	During pregnancy or up to 6 months after pregnancy	11	65		Age	4.28	1.69	34 ± 3.7	34 ± 7.7		5

9	Moller et al.	2013	Cancer registration dataset for the England population	Cohort	OS		Pregnancy 0–1 year before cancer diagnosis (moving window)	306	16,222	All	Cox regression for TNM available					11 years (maximum)	6
10	Zhou et al.	2014	University of Texas MD Anderson Cancer Center	Case-control	OS	41	During pregnancy or up to 6 months after pregnancy	18	18	1, 3, 4	Stage, age, Breslow's depth, ulceration, mitotic rate	1.63	2	30	31	Median 37.6 months (range, 3.8–96.5 months)	4
11	Johansson et al.	2014	National Swedish Cancer Registry	Cohort	DSS	6,857	Diagnosed within 9 months before or within 2 years after a delivery	1,019	5,838	IA, IB, II, and III–IV	Cox regression for age available			31	34.7	10 years (maximum)	6
12	Stensheim et al.	2009	Cancer Registry of Norway	Cohort	DSS	4,620	During pregnancy	160	4,460	All	Cox regression for age and TNM available	Not reported, no difference between	NR, no difference between	29	39	11.9 years	5
13	Travers et al.	1995	Massachusetts General Hospital Pigmented Lesion Clinic	Cohort	OS	465	During pregnancy or within the first year postpartum	45	420			2.28	1.22	31.8	33.2	1,963, 1,999 days	6

(Continued)

TABLE 7.3.1 Summary of the 17 Studies Included in the Systematic Review (cont.)

No.	Study	Year	Place	Design	Outcome	Total number of patients in the study	Melanoma diagnosis in relation to pregnancy (PAM definition in each study)	Number of PAM cases	Number of MM controls	Stage	Matching	Breslow's thickness, PAM (mm)	Breslow's thickness, MM (mm)	Mean age, PAM (years)	Mean age, MM (years)	Mean*, follow-up time (years)	NOS scoring
14	Daryanani et al.	2003	University Medical Center Groningen	Case–control	OS, DSS	2,567	During pregnancy	46	368		Age, post hoc NS for subtype, thickness, vascular invasion	2	1.7	30	36	Median 109 months	5
15	Silipo et al.	2006	Dermatological Institute, Rome	Case–control	OS, DSS	40	During pregnancy	10	30	All	Age, localization, histotype, and stage of melanoma	1.08	0.84	32 (28–35)		5 years	5
16	Houghton et al.	1981	Connecticut Tumour Registry	Case–control	OS	187	During pregnancy	12	175 (24 matched)	All	Age, anatomic site of primary melanoma, and stage			31.6	31.2	5 years	4
17	Sutherland et al.	1983	Tulane University School of Medicine	Case–control	OS	30	During pregnancy	18	12	1.2				27.5	25.6	5 years	4

DSS, Disease-specific survival; MM, malignant melanoma; NOS, Newcastle–Ottawa scoring; OS, overall survival; PAM, pregnancy-associated malignant melanoma; TNM, tumor node metastasis.

Study or subgroup	Weight	Hazard ratio Exp[(O – E)/V], Fixed, 95% CI	Hazard ratio Exp[(O – E)/V], fixed, 95% CI
Daryanani et al. [13] 2003	2.3%	0.73 [0.31, 1.70]	
Johansson et al. [11] 2014	33.5%	1.03 [0.83, 1.29]	
Lens et al. [14] 2004	13.9%	1.17 [0.83, 1.66]	
MacKie et al. [15] 1991	8.7%	1.14 [0.73, 1.77]	
McManamny et al. [16] 1989	1.7%	1.73 [0.64, 4.64]	
Miller et al. [17] 2010	0.2%	19.61 [0.95, 403.62]	
Moller et al. [3] 2013	11.9%	2.06 [1.42, 3.01]	
O'Meara et al. [18] 2005	7.4%	0.69 [0.43, 1.12]	
Reintgen et al. [19] 1985	4.9%	1.40 [0.78, 2.52]	
Silipo et al. [24] 2006	0.2%	1.56 [0.11, 21.45]	
Slingluff et al. [20] 1990	4.8%	1.35 [0.75, 2.44]	
Travers et al. [21] 1995	3.8%	1.31 [0.68, 2.55]	
Wong et al. [22] 1989	5.2%	1.14 [0.65, 2.02]	
Zhou et al. [23] 2014	1.5%	0.77 [0.27, 2.20]	
Total (95% CI)	100.0%	1.17 [1.03, 1.33]	
Tolal events			

Heterogeneity: $\chi^2 = 21.05$, df = 13 ($P = .07$); $I^2 = 38\%$
Test for overall effect: $Z = 2.38$ ($P = .02$)

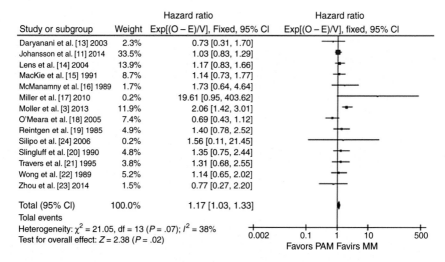

FIGURE 7.3.1 **Overall survival.** Patients with pregnancy-associated malignant melanoma (*PAM*) versus female patients with malignant melanoma (*MM*).

Study for subgroup	PAM Events	PAM Total	Melanoma Events	Melanoma Total	O – E	Variance	Weight	Peto odds ratio Exp [(O – E)/V], fixed, 95% CI	Peto odds ratio Exp [(O – E)/V], fixed, 95% CI
Daryanani et al. [13] 2003	10	46	77	368	0.23	8.59	12.3%	1.03 [0.53, 2.00]	
MacKie et al. [15] 1991	37	92	73	296	9.51	19.89	28.5%	1.61 [1.04, 2.50]	
Reintgen et al. [19] 1985	22	58	171	585	10.04	23.92	34.2%	1.52 [1.02, 2.27]	
Slingluff et al. [20] 1990	49	100	28	85	8.66	17.5	25.0%	1.64 [1.03, 2.62]	
Total (95% CI)		296		1334			100.0%	1.50 [1.19, 1.90]	
Total events	118		349						

Heterogeneity: $\chi^2 = 1.48$, df = 3 ($P = .69$); $I^2 = 0\%$
Test for overall effect: $Z = 3.40$ ($P = .0007$)

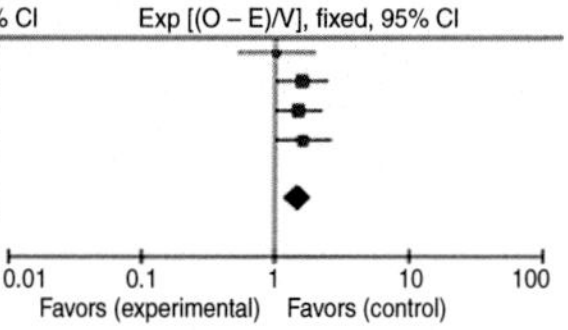

FIGURE 7.3.2 **Disease-free survival.** Patients with pregnancy-associated malignant melanoma (*PAM*) versus female patients with malignant melanoma (*MM*).

- In the DSS analysis, only two studies were included [11,25] and the results were expectedly not significant (total HR = 1.12, 95% CI: 0.92–1.36, *P* = .24).

2.1.1 *Limitations–Sensitivity Analyses*

- A number of sensitivity analyses were utilized to overcome a number of limitations. The most important examined the *effect of thickness—stage on the total outcome.*
- The total HR was significant (HR = 1.36; exp[(O − E)/V], fixed, 95% CI: 1.14–1.63; Fig. 7.3.3) with low heterogeneity ($I^2 = 10\%$, $P = .35$). Since this analysis is adjusted for stage and thickness, it could be the one with the greatest external validity.
- Heterogeneity was small to moderate in all analyses. Publication bias was examined via funnel plot and Egger's test was found to be not significant (Figs. 7.3.4–7.3.7).

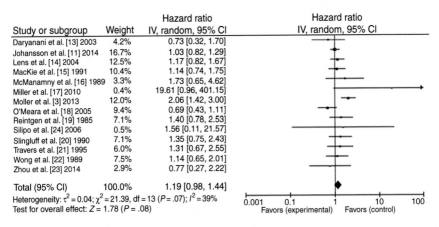

Study or subgroup	Weight	Hazard ratio IV, random, 95% CI
Daryanani et al. [13] 2003	4.2%	0.73 [0.32, 1.70]
Johansson et al. [11] 2014	16.7%	1.03 [0.82, 1.29]
Lens et al. [14] 2004	12.5%	1.17 [0.82, 1.67]
MacKie et al. [15] 1991	10.4%	1.14 [0.74, 1.75]
McManamny et al. [16] 1989	3.3%	1.73 [0.65, 4.62]
Miller et al. [17] 2010	0.4%	19.61 [0.96, 401.15]
Moller et al. [3] 2013	12.0%	2.06 [1.42, 3.00]
O'Meara et al. [18] 2005	9.4%	0.69 [0.43, 1.11]
Reintgen et al. [19] 1985	7.1%	1.40 [0.78, 2.53]
Silipo et al. [24] 2006	0.5%	1.56 [0.11, 21.57]
Slingluff et al. [20] 1990	7.1%	1.35 [0.75, 2.43]
Travers et al. [21] 1995	6.0%	1.31 [0.67, 2.55]
Wong et al. [22] 1989	7.5%	1.14 [0.65, 2.01]
Zhou et al. [23] 2014	2.9%	0.77 [0.27, 2.22]
Total (95% CI)	100.0%	1.19 [0.98, 1.44]

Heterogeneity: $\tau^2 = 0.04$; $\chi^2 = 21.39$, df = 13 ($P = .07$); $I^2 = 39\%$
Test for overall effect: $Z = 1.78$ ($P = .08$)

FIGURE 7.3.3   **Sensitivity analysis: use of random effects model, inverse variance.** Overall survival. Patients with pregnancy-associated malignant melanoma (*PAM*) versus female patients with malignant melanoma (*MM*).

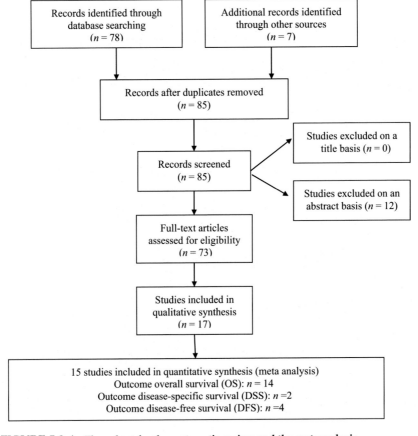

FIGURE 7.3.4   **Flow chart for the systematic review and the metaanalysis.**

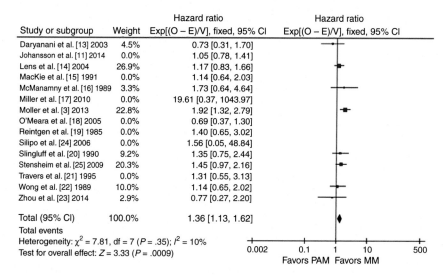

Study or subgroup	Weight	Hazard ratio Exp[(O – E)/V], fixed, 95% CI	Hazard ratio Exp[(O – E)/V], fixed, 95% CI
Daryanani et al. [13] 2003	4.5%	0.73 [0.31, 1.70]	
Johansson et al. [11] 2014	0.0%	1.05 [0.78, 1.41]	
Lens et al. [14] 2004	26.9%	1.17 [0.83, 1.66]	
MacKie et al. [15] 1991	0.0%	1.14 [0.64, 2.03]	
McManamny et al. [16] 1989	3.3%	1.73 [0.64, 4.64]	
Miller et al. [17] 2010	0.0%	19.61 [0.37, 1043.97]	
Moller et al. [3] 2013	22.8%	1.92 [1.32, 2.79]	
O'Meara et al. [18] 2005	0.0%	0.69 [0.37, 1.30]	
Reintgen et al. [19] 1985	0.0%	1.40 [0.65, 3.02]	
Silipo et al. [24] 2006	0.0%	1.56 [0.05, 48.84]	
Slingluff et al. [20] 1990	9.2%	1.35 [0.75, 2.44]	
Stensheim et al. [25] 2009	20.3%	1.45 [0.97, 2.16]	
Travers et al. [21] 1995	0.0%	1.31 [0.55, 3.13]	
Wong et al. [22] 1989	10.0%	1.14 [0.65, 2.02]	
Zhou et al. [23] 2014	2.9%	0.77 [0.27, 2.20]	
Total (95% CI)	100.0%	1.36 [1.13, 1.62]	

Total events
Heterogeneity: $\chi^2 = 7.81$, df = 7 ($P = .35$); $I^2 = 10\%$
Test for overall effect: $Z = 3.33$ ($P = .0009$)

0.002 0.1 1 10 500
Favors PAM Favors MM

FIGURE 7.3.5 **Sensitivity analysis: stensheim reporting DSS also included.** Studies that did not report on matching of stage and/or thickness are excluded (O'Meara, McKie, Miller, Reintgen, Travers and Johansson). Adjusted HRs for Moller and Sthensheim are used. Overall and disease-specific survival. Patients with pregnancy associated malignant melanoma (PAM) versus female patients with malignant melanoma (MM).

Study or subgroup	Weight	Hazard ratio IV, random, 95% CI	Hazard ratio IV, random, 95% CI
Daryanani et al. [13] 2003	4.6%	0.73 [0.32, 1.70]	
Johansson et al. [11] 2014	0.0%	1.05 [0.85, 1.30]	
Lens et al. [14] 2004	26.2%	1.17 [0.82, 1.67]	
MacKie et al. [15] 1991	0.0%	1.14 [0.65, 2.01]	
McManamny et al. [16] 1989	3.4%	1.73 [0.65, 4.62]	
Miller et al. [17] 2010	0.0%	19.61 [0.37, 1035.64]	
Moller et al. [3] 2013	23.5%	1.92 [1.33, 2.79]	
O'Meara et al. [18] 2005	0.0%	0.69 [0.37, 1.29]	
Reintgen et al. [19] 1985	0.0%	1.40 [0.65, 3.04]	
Silipo et al. [24] 2006	0.5%	1.56 [0.11, 21.57]	
Slingluff et al. [20] 1990	9.4%	1.35 [0.75, 2.44]	
Stensheim et al. [25] 2009	19.3%	1.45 [0.96, 2.18]	
Travers et al. [21] 1995	0.0%	1.31 [0.55, 3.14]	
Wong et al. [22] 1989	10.1%	1.14 [0.65, 2.01]	
Zhou et al. [23] 2014	2.9%	0.77 [0.27, 2.22]	
Total (95% CI)	100.0%	1.36 [1.14, 1.63]	

Heterogeneity: $\tau^2 = .00$; $\chi^2 = 7.87$, df = 8 ($P = .45$); $I^2 = 0\%$
Test for overall effect: $Z = 3.34$ ($P = .0008$)

0.01 0.1 1 10 100
Favors (experimental) Favors (control)

FIGURE 7.3.6 **Sensitivity analysis: stensheim reporting DSS also included.** Studies that did not report on matching of stage and/or thickness are excluded (O'Meara, McKie, Miller, Reintgen, Travers and Johansson). Adjusted HRs for Moller and Stensheim are used. Overall and disease-specific survival. Inverse variance with random effects. Patients with pregnancy associated malignant melanoma (PAM) versus female patients with malignant melanoma (MM).

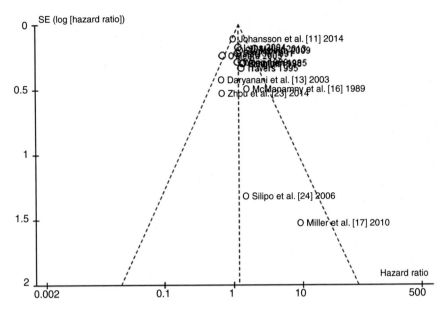

FIGURE 7.3.7   **Funnel plot of studies included in the meta-analysis.**

2.2 Sentinel Lymph Node Biopsy (SLNB) in Pregnant Women

- In a case series, SLNB was performed safely during pregnancy without adverse effects to the mothers and fetuses [26].
  - In general, SLNB can be performed in pregnant patients, with safety [27–30].
- During pregnancy, most experience with the SLNB technique has been gained in the field of breast cancer. The SLNB technique for breast cancer is safe during pregnancy and has not been reported to increase risk of malformation and fetal death [29].
- Notably, any procedure in pregnant women needs to be properly justified and based on adequate evidence. However, there is probably not sufficient evidence to justify SLNB in general [31], thus even more for pregnant patients.

3 DISCUSSION

- Currently available evidence suggests that PAM is associated with a worse prognosis than melanoma not related to pregnancy, in terms of both OS and DFS.
  - This finding is novel, since, up-to-date, such an association has not been established on the basis of a quantitative metaanalytical approach [7–9,32].

- The results of previous studies were inconsistent, with some of them suggesting that pregnancy worsens melanoma prognosis and some others failing to demonstrate such an association.
- These controversial data lead experts to conclude that existing evidence is insufficient to establish any impact of pregnancy on melanoma prognosis.
- The increased thickness of PAM, reported in several studies, was mainly attributed to a delayed diagnosis, which possibly results from the belief that nevi normally change during pregnancy. This leads to an underestimation of clinical characteristics that should be otherwise assessed as worrisome. Accordingly, the overall suggestion was that the management of PAM should be similar to melanoma not related to pregnancy, with the exception of some steps during the staging process, which should be avoided during pregnancy or postponed until delivery. Concerning the continuance of pregnancy after PAM diagnosis, the suggestion was that it should be discussed only on a social basis, taking into consideration the prognosis as determined by the disease stage.
- On the background of the unresolved controversy on the possible effect of pregnancy on melanoma prognosis, the latter [12] results might be highly relevant from a clinical aspect. Via a combination of the results from older studies that did not achieve to document a significant association between pregnancy and melanoma mortality, along with the results from recent studies, we were able to establish an unfavorable prognosis for melanoma diagnosed during pregnancy, a small but significant survival difference for both OS and DSS, favoring melanoma controls compared to PAM patients. For OS, this result is a 17% increased probability of mortality for PAM patients, which spans between 3 and 33%. For DFS, the result is a 50% increased probability of disease recurrence for PAM patients, which spans between 19 and 90%. The heterogeneity among studies included in the current metaanalysis was low for DFS ($P = .69$) and moderate ($P = .07$) for OS.
  - Clinicians dealing with PAM patients should take into consideration that existing evidence suggests a worse prognosis, compared to nonpregnant melanoma patients.
  - While this certainly justifies a very close and careful monitoring, no evidence indicates that early termination of pregnancy could improve the prognosis of the patient. Subsequently, the current strategy of discussing the pregnancy continuance on a social and family basis remains the optimal approach.
- Given the previous discussion, it should be emphasized that the only safe strategy to reduce PAM-related mortality is early diagnosis. Clinicians should be aware of the risk of missing melanoma because of the general belief that a changing mole during pregnancy is a normal finding. In this context, the usefulness of dermoscopy in evaluating pigmented skin lesions of pregnant women is unquestionable, and

the detection of even one melanoma criterion should immediately warrant excision.
- In conclusion, with the current systematic review we provide evidence that PAM is associated with a worse prognosis, compared to melanoma not related to pregnancy.

Take-home messages:

- Melanoma is the most common malignancy diagnosed during pregnancy.
- Pregnant women diagnosed with melanoma have a worse prognosis compared to nonpregnant women of similar demographics and staging.
- Increased clinician awareness is needed for changing moles during pregnancy.

References

[1] Lens M, Rosdahl I, Newton-Bishop J. Cutaneous melanoma during pregnancy: is the controversy over? J Clin Oncol 2009;27(19):e11–2. [author reply e13–4].
[2] Bannister-Tyrrell M, Roberts CL, Hasovits C, Nippita T, Ford JB. Incidence and outcomes of pregnancy-associated melanoma in New South Wales 1994–2008. Aust N Z J Obstet Gynaecol 2015;55:116–22.
[3] Moller H, Purushotham A, Linklater KM, et al. Recent childbirth is an adverse prognostic factor in breast cancer and melanoma, but not in Hodgkin lymphoma. Eur J Cancer 2013;49(17):3686–93.
[4] Paradela S, Fonseca E, Pita-Fernandez S, et al. Melanoma under 18 years and pregnancy: report of three cases. Eur J Dermatol 2010;20(2):186–8.
[5] Youn SH, Lee YW, Seung NR, et al. Rapidly progressing malignant melanoma influenced by pregnancy. Int J Dermatol 2010;49(11):1318–20.
[6] Maleka A, Enblad G, Sjors G, Lindqvist A, Ullenhag GJ. Treatment of metastatic malignant melanoma with vemurafenib during pregnancy. J Clin Oncol 2013;31(11):e192–3.
[7] Gupta A, Driscoll MS. Do hormones influence melanoma? Facts and controversies. Clin Dermatol 2010;28(3):287–92.
[8] Jhaveri MB, Driscoll MS, Grant-Kels JM. Melanoma in pregnancy. Clin Obstet Gynecol 2011;54(4):537–45.
[9] Peccatori FA, Azim HA Jr, Orecchia R, et al. Cancer, pregnancy and fertility: ESMO clinical practice guidelines for diagnosis, treatment and follow-up. Ann Oncol 2013;24(Suppl. 6):vi160–70.
[10] Enninga EA, Holtan SG, Creedon DJ, et al. Immunomodulatory effects of sex hormones: requirements for pregnancy and relevance in melanoma. Mayo Clinic Proc 2014;89(4):520–35.
[11] Johansson AL, Andersson TM, Plym A, Ullenhag GJ, Moller H, Lambe M. Mortality in women with pregnancy-associated malignant melanoma. J Am Acad Dermatol 2014;71(6):1093–101.
[12] Kyrgidis A, Lallas A, Moscarella E, Longo C, Alfano R, Argenziano G. Does pregnancy influence melanoma prognosis? A meta-analysis. Melanoma Res 2017. doi: 10.1097/CMR.0000000000000334 [Epub ahead of print].
[13] Daryanani D, Plukker JT, De Hullu JA, Kuiper H, Nap RE, Hoekstra HJ. Pregnancy and early-stage melanoma. Cancer 2003;97(9):2248–53.

[14] Lens MB, Rosdahl I, Ahlbom A, et al. Effect of pregnancy on survival in women with cutaneous malignant melanoma. J Clin Oncol 2004;22(21):4369–75.

[15] MacKie RM, Bufalino R, Morabito A, Sutherland C, Cascinelli N. Lack of effect of pregnancy on outcome of melanoma. For The World Health Organisation Melanoma Programme. Lancet 1991;337(8742):653–5.

[16] McManamny DS, Moss ALH, Briggs JC, Pocock PV. Melanoma and pregnancy: a long-term follow-up. Br J Obstet Gynaecol 1989;96(12):1419–23.

[17] Miller E, Barnea Y, Gur E, et al. Malignant melanoma and pregnancy: second thoughts. J Plast Reconstr Aesthet Surg 2010;63(7):1163–8.

[18] O'Meara AT, Cress R, Xing G, Danielsen B, Smith LH. Malignant melanoma in pregnancy. Cancer 2005;103(6):1217–26.

[19] Reintgen DS, McCarty KS, Vollmer R, Cox E, Seigler HF. Malignant melanoma and pregnancy. Cancer 1985;55(6):1340–4.

[20] Slingluff CLJ, Reintgen DS, Vollmer RT, Seigler HF. Malignant melanoma arising during pregnancy: a study of 100 patients. Ann Surg 1990;211(5):552–9.

[21] Travers RL, Sober AJ, Berwick M, Mihm MC, Harnhill RL, Duncan LM. Increased thickness of pregnancy-associated melanoma. Br J Dermatol 1995;132(6):876–83.

[22] Wong JH, Sterns EE, Kopald KH, Nizze JA, Morton DL. Prognostic significance of pregnancy in stage I melanoma. Arch Surg 1989;124(10):1227–30. [discussion 1230–1].

[23] Zhou JH, Kim KB, Myers JN, et al. Immunohistochemical expression of hormone receptors in melanoma of pregnant women, nonpregnant women, and men. Am J Dermatopathol 2014;36(1):74–9.

[24] Silipo V, De Simone P, Mariani G, Buccini P, Ferrari A, Catricala C. Malignant melanoma and pregnancy. Melanoma Res 2006;16(6):497–500.

[25] Stensheim H, Moller B, van Dijk T, Fossa SD. Cause-specific survival for women diagnosed with cancer during pregnancy or lactation: a registry-based cohort study. J Clin Oncol 2009;27(1):45–51.

[26] Andtbacka RH, Donaldson MR, Bowles TL, et al. Sentinel lymph node biopsy for melanoma in pregnant women. Ann Surg Oncol 2013;20(2):689–96.

[27] Broer N, Buonocore S, Goldberg C, et al. A proposal for the timing of management of patients with melanoma presenting during pregnancy. J Surg Oncol 2012;106(1):36–40.

[28] Chakera AH, Hesse B, Burak Z, et al. EANM-EORTC general recommendations for sentinel node diagnostics in melanoma. Eur J Nucl Med Mol Imaging 2009;36(10):1713–42.

[29] Gziri MM, Han SN, Amant F. Use of general anesthesia and sentinel node procedure during pregnancy. J Surg Oncol 2012;106(8):1008.

[30] Marsden JR, Newton-Bishop JA, Burrows L, et al. Revised U.K. guidelines for the management of cutaneous melanoma 2010. Br J Dermatol 2010;163(2):238–56.

[31] Kyrgidis A, Tzellos T, Mocellin S, et al. Sentinel lymph node biopsy followed by lymph node dissection for localised primary cutaneous melanoma. Cochrane Database Syst Rev 2015;5. CD010307.

[32] Lens M, Bataille V. Melanoma in relation to reproductive and hormonal factors in women: current review on controversial issues. Cancer Causes Control 2008;19(5):437–42.

7.4

Pediatric Melanoma and Atypical Spitz Tumor

Elvira Moscarella*,**, *Gabriella Brancaccio**

*University of Campania Luigi Vanvitelli, Naples, Italy
**Arcispedale S. Maria Nuova, IRCCS, Reggio Emilia, Italy

1 INTRODUCTION

- Melanoma incidence is very low in the pediatric age group (patients from 0 to 18 years of age).
  - The studies available in the literature are not uniform in inclusion criteria for age. Despite the varying age cutoffs, it seems to be clear that significant differences in terms of histological subtype of melanoma, incidence, and mortality rates exist between children (prepubertal cases, 0–12 years) and adolescents and young adults (>12 years).
    - Younger patients have lower melanoma incidence and higher survival rate as compared to older ones. Their melanomas are more frequently of the nodular subtype with higher Breslow's thickness at diagnosis.
- Staging and follow-up recommendations do not differ from adult patients in the majority of available guidelines, with the exception of the recently published NICE guidelines that suggest slightly different imaging procedures for younger patients.
- One major problem in the diagnosis and management of melanocytic lesions in this age group is related to the higher incidence of spitzoid melanocytic neoplasms.
  - Atypical Spitz tumors (ASTs) are difficult-to-diagnose melanocytic lesions from a clinical and histopathological point of view. Incidence of AST is higher in children and young adults as compared to that in older patients. They have a tendency for locoregional spread, with an overall high survival rate.

2 PEDIATRIC MELANOMA

2.1 Incidence

In children under 15 years of age the incidence of malignant melanoma is found to be about 0.7–0.8 per million in the United States. The incidence in individuals aged 15–19 is reported to be more than 10 per million.

2.2 Clinical and Dermoscopic Diagnosis

Due to its rarity, little is known about the clinical appearance of pediatric melanoma.

Summarizing the currently available knowledge, the following scenarios have to be taken into consideration:

1. *Peculiar clinical appearance seems to characterize childhood melanoma.*
   a. Several reports describe specific characteristics of childhood melanoma including thicker lesions, nodular histotype, advanced stage, and amelanotic tumors (especially for patients under the age of 10 years).
   b. Modified ABCD detection criteria for melanoma have been suggested, as conventional criteria lack in melanoma of the younger age. Instead, features such as amelanosis, bleeding, raised papulonodular primary lesions, and de novo development (not in association with a preexisting nevus) are observed.
   c. Interestingly, the most common prebiopsy diagnosis for amelanotic lesions was pyogenic granuloma.
      - Management strategy: Melanoma screening in young children is not recommended, given the rarity of the disease. Attention should be paid on large, ulcerated, rapidly growing, nodular lesions. Excision and histopathological examination is mandatory in these cases, keeping in mind that the main clinical and dermoscopic differential diagnosis of melanoma in children is not dysplastic or Clark's nevi but rather spitzoid melanocytic lesions (Spitz nevus and AST, see the subsequent text), and banal nonmelanocytic lesions, such as angioma or pyogenic granuloma. No clear-cut criteria are available for the clinical and dermoscopic differential diagnosis of pyogenic granuloma from melanoma and AST (Fig. 7.4.1).
2. *Conventional melanoma features seem more likely to be found in adolescents and young adults.*
   a. After puberty, the total number of nevus count is rising. In this scenario, differential diagnosis of melanoma may include atypical nevi. Again, melanoma screening is not routinely recommended.

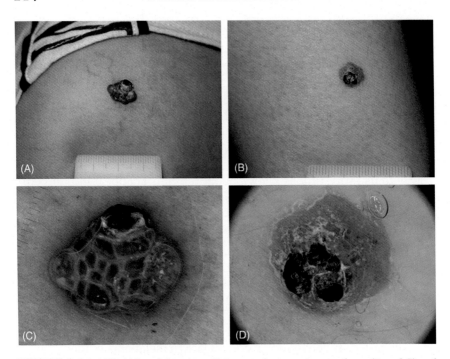

FIGURE 7.4.1 **Clinical and dermoscopic image of pyogenic granuloma (A and C) and atypical Spitz tumor (B and D).** (A) Amelanotic, ulcerated nodule arising on the shoulder of a 9-year-old boy. The lesion was reported as rapidly growing. (B) Amelanotic, ulcerated nodule arising on the leg of an 8-year-old girl. (C) Under dermoscopy, red lacunas separated by white septa are detected; ulceration is visible as a brown to black blotch. (D) Dermoscopically, the lesion presents a nonspecific pattern; a pink background coloration, white lines, and ulceration are visible.

This should be considered in cases of high total nevus count and additional risk factors, such as family history of melanoma and fair skin type (Fig. 7.4.2)

Management strategy: Periodic clinical and dermoscopic examination is warranted in these cases. However, physiological changes and "volatility" of nevi in children have to be carefully considered in the decision-making process. Efficacy of melanoma detection in children and adolescents was demonstrated to be lower than in adults in recent studies. A study based on a 10-year period database of excised melanocytic lesions in children used the number needed to excise (NNE) value to evaluate the efficacy of melanoma screening (obtained dividing the total number of excised lesions by the number of melanomas). The NNE value for pediatric population (0–18 years) was 20 times higher than the rates usually found in adult patients. This means

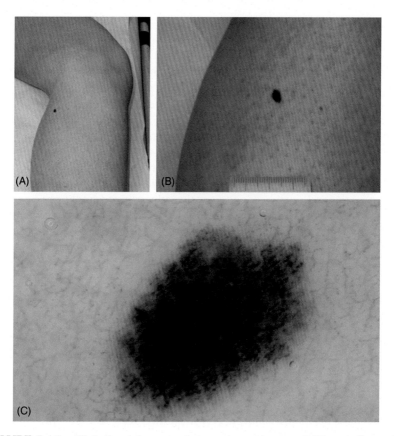

FIGURE 7.4.2 **Clinical and dermoscopic appearance of a superficial spreading melanoma, 0.3 mm Breslow's thickness, in a 17-year-old girl.** Clinical aspect (A) and close-up (B) of the lesion. The patient had fair skin type, multiple nevi, and family history of melanoma. (C) Under dermoscopy atypical network is detected, composed of thick, dark brown to black lines with abrupt ending.

that a very high number of benign nevi (i.e., approximately 594) were excised to detect 1 melanoma. Similar data were reported by a later analysis.

3. *The risk of melanoma arising on small- to medium-sized congenital nevi (CMN) is a matter of debate.*

   a. CMN are classified and divided into four groups based on the largest expected adult diameter, in centimeters:

   – Small, <1.5 cm
   – Medium (M1: 1.5–10 cm, M2: >10–20 cm)
   – Large (L1: 20–30 cm, L2: 30–40 cm)
   – Giant (G1: 40–60 cm, G2: >60 cm)

The risk of melanoma development within small and medium CMN is a matter of debate. Based on current data, this risk seems to be less than 1% over a lifetime. In three large cohort studies of patients with a small or medium CMN who were followed for a mean of 13.5 years (n = 680 patients; mean age at entry ~10 years), no melanomas were observed.

- Management strategy: In general, if no atypical clinical and dermoscopic features are detected, these nevi can be managed on an individual basis and monitored or excised based on patient compliance to follow-up and cosmetic concerns of parents and patients. In general, excision of medium-sized CMN can be proposed to be performed after puberty. Alternatively, clinical follow-up should be scheduled annually for these lesions, and digital clinical dermoscopic imaging can be performed to detect early changes (Fig. 7.4.3).

4. *A multidisciplinary approach is required for the management of large/giant CMN.*

   a. The lifetime risk of melanoma (cutaneous or extracutaneous) associated with a large or giant CMN is thought to be less than 5%. Melanoma risk is higher in patients with CMN that have a projected adult size of more than 40–60 cm in diameter. Additional risk factors for melanoma include a truncal location and numerous (e.g., N20) satellite nevi.

   b. Approximately half of melanomas in patients with a large or giant CMN are diagnosed during the first 5 years of life. Misinterpretation of proliferative nodules with atypical histological findings as melanoma may occur in this age group.

   c. Neurocutaneous melanocytosis (NCM) represents proliferation of melanocytes in the central nervous system (CNS) in addition to the skin in patients with CMN. The presence of numerous CMN, regardless of whether or not there is a large or giant CMN, represents the strongest risk factor for NCM. NCM is divided into symptomatic and asymptomatic forms, with brain involvement detected via MRI screening in the latter group. MRI findings of NCM can be present in the brain parenchyma, and can include obvious masses and gadolinium enhancement of diffusely thickened meninges (associated with a worse prognosis). Recent studies have drawn attention to spinal abnormalities such as tethered cord, intraspinal lipoma, and arachnoid cysts in patients with large/giant CMN. Nowadays, we speak about "congenital melanocytic nevus syndrome" to indicate the spectrum of CNS abnormalities described in

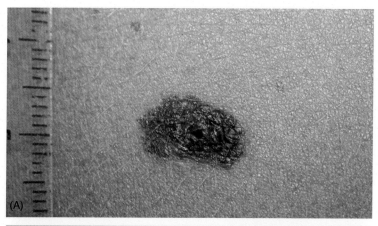

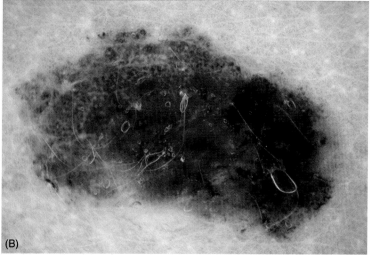

FIGURE 7.4.3 **Superficial spreading melanoma arising on a small congenital nevus in an 11-year-old boy.** (A) Clinically, the lesion is a dark brown macule presenting an asymmetric, eccentric, and slightly palpable blue to black area. (B) In dermoscopy, a typical cobblestone pattern is detected on side of the lesion. The elevated part of the lesion is characterized by a blue-white veil and irregular black blotches.

association with CMN. Approximately 4% of patients with high-risk CMN develop symptomatic NCM, which has a poor prognosis even in the absence of melanoma.

— Management strategy: Melanomas that arise within large and giant CMN more often develop deep in the dermis or in the subcutaneous tissue, which can make early detection difficult.

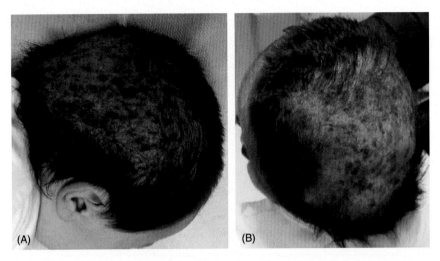

FIGURE 7.4.4 **Giant congenital nevus of the scalp in a 3-month-old girl.** The lesion was present since birth. The lesion was composed of a hairy nevus and multiple, scattered, smaller nonhairy melanocytic lesions (A). In the occipital area (B).

The management of these patients should be multidisciplinary, including MRI imaging and neurological examination. For screening congenital neurological lesions, a single MRI in multiple CMN is a clinically relevant strategy. In case of stepwise change in neurological/developmental symptoms or signs, an MRI with contrast of the brain and spine should be considered to look for new CNS melanoma (Fig. 7.4.4).

2.3 Staging and Follow-Up

Staging and follow-up recommendations do not differ from adult patients in the majority of available guidelines, with the exception of the recently published NICE guidelines that suggest MRI instead of CT scan as imaging procedure for younger patients, especially for the diagnosis of suspected brain metastasis.

2.4 Treatment

Given the rarity of the disease in young people, prospective clinical trials tailored to children are not currently available and most adult treatment protocols are generally not accessible to children. Things are changing, however, and phase 1–2 trials with novel drugs, such as BRAF inhibitors and ipilimumab, are currently ongoing.

3 ATYPICAL SPITZ TUMOR

- ASTs are problematic melanocytic neoplasms displaying intermediate histopathological features between Spitz nevi and spitzoid melanoma, especially found in the younger age group, and carrying uncertain malignant potential.
- The exact clinicopathological definition of AST is a matter of ongoing debate among dermatopathologists, since the first description, by Smith and coworkers, in 1989. Nowadays, some opinion leaders do not accept the concept of a "gray zone" in dermatopathology, and are prone to classify spitzoid lesions as either benign (Spitz nevus) or malignant (spitzoid melanoma). Others suggest that spitzoid lesions are on a morphobiological spectrum ranging from benign to clear-cut malignant lesions, with AST placed in the middle of this spectrum. There remains a lack of consensus, with diagnostic agreement among dermatopathologists significantly lower than for nonspitzoid melanocytic neoplasms, especially with regard to prediction of outcome.
- There are no reliable histological criteria that allow a histopathological identification of AST with aggressive behavior, with relevant subsequent management problems for the clinicians.

3.1 Clinical and Dermoscopic Diagnosis

A recent study examined the clinical and dermoscopic aspect of a series of AST, collected retrospectively in a multicenter study, and compared with a series of Spitz nevi. The results of the study showed that:

- AST tend to present more frequently as nodular lesions.
- The main dermoscopic patterns of AST are the multicomponent and nonspecific patterns.
- Both amelanotic AST and Spitz nevi may present under dermoscopy dotted vessels and white lines (Fig. 7.4.5).

3.2 Management

- Surgical excision with clear margins is recommended for AST.
- When a diagnosis of AST is suspected histologically, revision by a panel of expert dermatopathologists is strongly suggested. Additionally, molecular biology testing might be considered, even if the accuracy and the limits of these techniques have not been widely elucidated.
- Identifying molecular markers of AST with aggressive behavior represents an important goal, with promising methods including

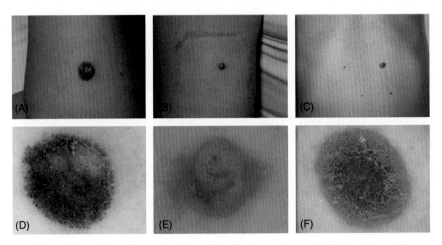

FIGURE 7.4.5 **Clinical (A–C) and dermoscopic (D–F) images of atypical Spitz tumors.** (A) A pigmented nodule arising on the arm of an 8-year-old girl. (B) An amelanotic nodule on the arm of a 6-year-old girl. (C) An amelanotic nodule on the abdomen of an 18-year-old boy. (D) Dermoscopy revealing a multicomponent pattern, composed of irregular brown to black globules, milky-red areas, and central blue pigmentation. (E) Dermoscopy revealing a nonspecific pattern, with pink to white background color and dotted and irregular vessels. (F) Under dermoscopy, pink color, dotted vessels, and white lines are detected.

array-based comparative genomic hybridization and fluorescence in situ hybridization (FISH) probes. Recent studies have found that specific genomic alterations (e.g., homozygous 9p21 deletions; 6p25 or 11q13 gains) are associated with aggressive clinical behavior of ASTs. In contrast, isolated deletions in 6q23 confer a favorable prognosis.

3.3 Sentinel Lymph Node Biopsy

- The decision to perform a sentinel lymph node biopsy should be considered in the light of the recent evidence on the absence of prognostic value of this technique. The best available evidence on the topic is a recent systematic review in which 541 patients with AST were included in the study. AST was associated with sentinel lymph node metastasis in more than 30% of cases (a value higher than in melanoma); however, 535 patients (99%) had a favorable prognosis.
- Existing data do not show any prognostic benefit of sentinel lymph node biopsy in patients with ASTs. However, the lack of high-quality evidence must be taken into account when interpreting these findings.
- Discussing all suspected atypical spitzoid lesions at the specialist skin cancer multidisciplinary team is highly recommended, as well as taking into account that sentinel lymph node biopsy, and the procedures after a possible positive result such as complete lymph

node dissection, is associated with high rates of morbidity, especially in children.

- It might be prudent to use complete excision with clear margins and careful clinical follow-up.
- FISH analysis could be useful to identify patients with more aggressive tumors, for which sentinel lymph node biopsy might have a therapeutic benefit.

3.4 Follow-Up

- No uniform guidelines exist on the better follow-up strategies for patients diagnosed with AST.
- Since the majority of recurrences are local or locoregional, a careful clinical follow-up seems to be the best strategy.
- Patients with more aggressive tumors, identified, for example, by FISH analysis, could benefit from lymph node ultrasound.
- Again, discussion at the specialist skin cancer multidisciplinary team is highly recommended.

Further Reading

Aldrink JH, Selim MA, Diesen DL, et al. Pediatric melanoma: a single-institution experience of 150 patients. J Pediatr Surg 2009;44:1514–21.

Alikhan AA, Ibrahimi OA, Eisen DB. Congenital melanocytic nevi: where are we now? Part I. Clinical presentation, epidemiology, pathogenesis, histology, malignant transformation, and neurocutaneous melanosis. J Am Acad Dermatol 2012;67:495.e1–495.e17.

Barnhill RL, Argenyi ZB, From L, et al. Atypical Spitz nevi/tumor: lack of consensus for diagnosis, discrimination from melanoma, and prediction of outcome. Hum Pathol 1999;30:513–20.

Barnhill RL, Flotte TJ, Fleischli M, et al. Cutaneous melanoma and atypical Spitz tumors in children. Cancer 1995;76:1833–45.

Barnhill RL, Kutzner H, Schmidt B, et al. Atypical spitzoid melanocytic neoplasms with angiotropism: a potential mechanism of locoregional involvement. Am J Dermatopathol 2011;33:236–43.

Berk DR, LaBuz E, Dadras SS, Johnson DL, Swetter SM. Melanoma and melanocytic tumors of uncertain malignant potential in children, adolescents and young adults—the Stanford experience 1995–2008. Pediatr Dermatol 2010;27:244–54.

Bett BJ. Large or multiple congenital melanocytic nevi: occurrence of cutaneous melanoma in 1008 persons. J Am Acad Dermatol 2005;52:793–7.

Bleyer AOLM, Barr R, Ries LA. Cancer epidemiology in older adolescents and young adults 15 to 29 years of age including SEER incidence and survival: 1975–2000. Bethesda: National Cancer Institute; 2006.

Brecht IB, Bremensdorfer C, Schneider DT, et al. Rare malignant pediatric tumors registered in the German Childhood Cancer Registry 2001–2010. Pediatr Blood Cancer 2014;61:1202–9.

Brecht IB, Garbe C, Gefeller O, et al. 443 paediatric cases of malignant melanoma registered with the German Central Malignant Melanoma Registry between 1983 and 2011. Eur J Cancer 2015;51(7):861–8.

Busam KJ, Murali R, Pulitzer M, et al. Atypical spitzoid melanocytic tumors with positive sentinel lymph nodes in children and teenagers, and comparison with histologically unambiguous and lethal melanomas. Am J Surg Pathol 2009;33:1386–95.

Carac C, Mozzillo N, Di Monta G, et al. Sentinel lymph node biopsy in atypical Spitz nevi: is it useful? Eur J Surg Oncol 2012;38:932–5.

Casso EM, Grin-Jorgensen CM, Grant-Kels JM. Spitz nevi. J Am Acad Dermatol 1992;27:901–13.

Ceballos PI, Ruiz-Maldonado R, Mihm MC Jr. Melanoma in children. N Engl J Med 1995;332:656–62.

Cerrato F, Wallins JS, Webb ML, McCarty ER, Schmidt BA, Labow BI. Outcomes in pediatric atypical Spitz tumors treated without sentinel lymph node biopsy. Pediatr Dermatol 2012;29:448–53.

Cerroni L, Barnhill R, Elder D, et al. Melanocytic tumors of uncertain malignant potential: results of a tutorial held at the XXIX symposium of the International Society of Dermatopathology in Graz, October 2008. Am J Surg Pathol 2010;34:314–26.

Cohen B. To biopsy or not to biopsy changing moles in children and adolescents: are we removing too many pigmented nevi in this age group? Arch Dermatol 2011;147:659–60.

Conti EM, Cercato MC, Gatta G, et al. Childhood melanoma in Europe since 1978: a population-based survival study. Eur J Cancer 2001;37:780–4.

Cordoro KM, Gupta D, Frieden IJ, et al. Pediatric melanoma: results of a large cohort study and proposal for modified ABCD detection criteria for children. J Am Acad Dermatol 2013;68:913–25.

Dawson HA, Atherton DJ, Mayou B. A prospective study of congenital melanocytic naevi: progress report and evaluation after 6 years. Br J Dermatol 1996;134:617–23.

de Maleissye MF, Beauchet A, Saiag P, et al. Sunscreen use and melanocytic nevi in children: a systematic review. Pediatr Dermatol 2013;30:51–9.

De Vries E, Steliarova-Foucher E, Spatz A, et al. Skin cancer incidence and survival in European children and adolescents (1978–1997). Report from the Automated Childhood Cancer Information System project. Eur J Cancer 2006;42:2170–82.

Downard CD, Rapkin LB, Gow KW. Melanoma in children and adolescents. Surg Oncol 2007;16:215–20.

Egan CL, Oliveria SA, Elenitsas R, et al. Cutaneous melanoma risk and phenotypic changes in large congenital nevi: a follow-up study of 46 patients. J Am Acad Dermatol 1998;39:923–32.

Ferrara G, Gianotti R, Cavicchini S, Salviato T, Zalaudek I, Argenziano G. Spitz nevus, Spitz tumor, and spitzoid melanoma: a comprehensive clinicopathologic overview. Dermatol Clin 2013;31:589–98. viii.

Ferrara G, Zalaudek I, Savarese I, et al. Pediatric atypical spitzoid neoplasms. A review with emphasis on 'red' ('Spitz') tumors and 'blue' ('Blitz') tumors. Dermatology 2010;220:306–10.

Ferrari A, Bisogno G, Cecchetto G, et al. Cutaneous melanoma in children and adolescents: the Italian rare tumors in pediatric age project experience. J Pediatr 2014;164:376–82. e2.

Ferrari A, Bono A, Baldi M, et al. Does melanoma behave differently in younger children than in adults? A retrospective study of 33 cases of childhood melanoma from a single institution. Pediatrics 2005;115:649–54.

Gallagher RP, Rivers JK, Lee TK, et al. Broad-spectrum sunscreen use and the development of new nevi in white children: a randomized controlled trial. JAMA 2000;283:2955–60.

Gamblin TC, Edington H, Kirkwood JM, Rao UNM. Sentinel lymph node biopsy for atypical melanocytic lesions with spitzoid features. Ann Surg Oncol 2006;13:1664–70.

Garbe C, Peris K, Hauschild A, et al. Diagnosis and treatment of melanoma. European consensus-based interdisciplinary guideline—update 2012. Eur J Cancer 2012;48:2375–90.

Gerami P, Scolyer RA, Xu X, et al. Risk assessment for atypical spitzoid melanocytic neo-plasms using FISH to identify chromosomal copy number aberrations. Am J Surg Pathol 2013;37:676–84.

Ghazi B, Carlson GW, Murray DR, et al. Utility of lymph node assessment for atypical spitzoid melanocytic neoplasms. Ann Surg Oncol 2010;17:2471–5.

Hale EK, Stein J, Ben-Porat L, et al. Association of melanoma and neurocutaneous melanocytosis with large congenital melanocytic naevi: results from the NYU-LCMN registry. Br J Dermatol 2005;152:512–7.

Han D, Zager JS, Han G, et al. The unique clinical characteristics of melanoma diagnosed in children. Ann Surg Oncol 2012;19:3888–95.

Hung T, Piris A, Lobo A, et al. Sentinel lymph node metastasis is not predictive of poor outcome in patients with problematic spitzoid melanocytic tumors. Hum Pathol 2013;44:87–94.

Ka VS, Dusza SW, Halpern AC, Marghoob AA. The association between large congenital melanocytic naevi and cutaneous melanoma: preliminary findings from an internet-based registry of 379 patients. Melanoma Res 2005;15:61–7.

Karlsson MA, Wahlgren CF, Wiklund K, Rodvall Y. Parental sun-protective regimens and prevalence of common melanocytic naevi among 7-year-old children in Sweden: changes over a 5-year period. Br J Dermatol 2011;164:830–7.

Karlsson PM, Fredrikson M. Cutaneous malignant melanoma in children and adolescents in Sweden, 1993–2002: the increasing trend is broken. Int J Cancer 2007;121:323–8.

Kelley SW, Cockerell CJ. Sentinel lymph node biopsy as an adjunct to management of histologically difficult to diagnose melanocytic lesions: a proposal. J Am Acad Dermatol 2000;42:527–30.

Kinsler VA, Birley J, Atherton DJ. Great Ormond Street Hospital for Children Registry for congenital melanocytic naevi: prospective study 1988–2007. Part 1—epidemiology, phenotype and outcomes. Br J Dermatol 2009;160:143–50.

Krengel S, Hauschild A, Schäfer T. Melanoma risk in congenital melanocytic naevi: a systematic review. Br J Dermatol 2006;155:1–8.

Krengel S, Scope A, Dusza SW, Vonthein R, Marghoob AA. New recommendations for the categorization of cutaneous features of congenital melanocytic nevi. J Am Acad Dermatol 2013;68:441–51.

Lallas A, Kyrgidis A, Ferrara G, et al. Atypical Spitz tumors and sentinel lymph node biopsy: a systematic review. Lancet Oncol 2014;15:e178.

Lange JR, Palis BE, Chang DC, et al. Melanoma in children and teenagers: an analysis of patients from the National Cancer Data Base. J Clin Oncol 2007;25:1363–8.

LeBoit PE. 'Safe' Spitz and its alternatives. Pediatr Dermatol 2002;19:163–5.

Leboit PE. What do these cells prove? Am J Dermatopathol 2003;25:355–6.

Lee TK, Rivers JK, Gallagher RP. Site-specific protective effect of broad-spectrum sunscreen on nevus development among white school-children in a randomized trial. J Am Acad Dermatol 2005;52:786–92.

Linabery AM, Ross JA. Trends in childhood cancer incidence in the U.S. (1992–2004). Cancer 2008;112:416–32.

Lohmann CM, Coit DG, Brady MS, Berwick M, Busam KJ. Sentinel lymph node biopsy in patients with diagnostically controversial spitzoid melanocytic tumors. Am J Surg Pathol 2002;26:47–55.

Ludgate MW, Fullen DR, Lee J, et al. The atypical Spitz tumor of uncertain biologic potential: a series of 67 patients from a single institution. Cancer 2009;115:631–41.

National Collaborating Centre for Cancer (UK). Melanoma: assessment and management. London, UK: National Institute for Health and Care Excellence; 2015.

Metzler G, Eigentler TK, Held L, et al. Molecular genetic classification of difficult melanocytic tumors. J Dtsch Dermatol Ges 2013;11(Suppl. 4):11–8.

Mones JM, Ackerman AB. "Atypical" Spitz's nevus, "malignant" Spitz's nevus, and "metastasizing" Spitz's nevus: a critique in historical perspective of three concepts flawed fatally. Am J Dermatopathol 2004;26:310–33.

Moore-Olufemi S, Herzog C, Warneke C, et al. Outcomes in pediatric melanoma: comparing prepubertal to adolescent pediatric patients. Ann Surg 2011;253:1211–5.

Moscarella E, Lallas A, Kyrgydis A, et al. Clinical and dermoscopic features of atypical Spitz tumors: a multicenter, retrospective, case–control study. J Am Acad Dermatol 2015;73:777–84.

Moscarella E, Piccolo V, Argenziano G, et al. Problematic lesions in children. Dermatol Clin 2013;31:535–47.

Moscarella E, Zalaudek I, Cerroni L, et al. Excised melanocytic lesions in children and adolescents—a 10-year survey. Br J Dermatol 2012;167:368–73.

Murali R, Sharma RN, Thompson JF, et al. Sentinel lymph node biopsy in histologically ambiguous melanocytic tumors with spitzoid features (so-called atypical spitzoid tumors). Ann Surg Oncol 2008;15:302–9.

Neuhold JC, Friesenhahn J, Gerdes N, Krengel S. Case reports of fatal or metastasizing melanoma in children and adolescents: a systematic analysis of the literature. Pediatr Dermatol 2015;32(1):13–22.

Oliveria SA, Saraiya M, Geller AC, et al. Sun exposure and risk of melanoma. Arch Dis Child 2006;91:131–8.

Oliveria SA, Selvam N, Mehregan D, et al. Biopsies of nevi in children and adolescents in the United States, 2009 through 2013. JAMA Dermatol 2015;151(4):447–8.

Pappo AS. Melanoma in children and adolescents. Eur J Cancer 2003;39:2651–61.

Paradela S, Fonseca E, Pita-Fernandez S, et al. Prognostic factors for melanoma in children and adolescents: a clinicopathologic, single-center study of 137 patients. Cancer 2010;116:4334–44.

Ries LA, Eisner MP, Kosary CL, et al. SEER cancer statistics review, 1973–1999. Bethesda: National Cancer Institute, SEER Program, NIH Pub.; 2002.

Roaten JB, Partrick DA, Pearlman N, Gonzalez RJ, Gonzalez R, McCarter MD. Sentinel lymph node biopsy for melanoma and other melanocytic tumors in adolescents. J Pediatr Surg 2005;40:232–5.

Ruiz-Maldonado R, Tamayo L, Laterza AM, Duran C. Giant pigmented nevi: clinical, histopathologic, and therapeutic considerations. J Pediatr 1992;120:906–11.

Sahin S, Levin L, Kopf AW, et al. Risk of melanoma in medium-sized congenital melanocytic nevi: a follow-up study. J Am Acad Dermatol 1998;39:428–33.

Sander B, Karlsson P, Rosdahl I, et al. Cutaneous malignant melanoma in Swedish children and teenagers 1973–1992: a clinico-pathological study of 130 cases. Int J Cancer 1999;80:646–51.

Schaffer JV. Update on melanocytic nevi in children. Clin Dermatol 2015;33(3):368–86.

Scope A, Dusza SW, Marghoob AA, et al. Clinical and dermoscopic stability and volatility of melanocytic nevi in a population-based cohort of children in Framingham school system. J Invest Dermatol 2011;131:1615–21.

Sepehr A, Chao E, Trefrey B, et al. Long-term outcome of Spitz-type melanocytic tumors. Arch Dermatol 2011;147:1173–9.

Smith A, Harrison S, Nowak M, Buettner P, Maclennan R. Changes in the pattern of sun exposure and sun protection in young children from tropical Australia. J Am Acad Dermatol 2013;68:774–83.

Smith KJ, Barrett TL, Skelton HG III, et al. Spindle cell and epithelioid cell nevi with atypia and metastasis (malignant Spitz nevus). Am J Surg Pathol 1989;13:931–9.

Spatz A, Calonje E, Handfield-Jones S, Barnhill RL. Spitz tumors in children: a grading system for risk stratification. Arch Dermatol 1999;135:282–5.

Strouse JJ, Fears TR, Tucker MA, et al. Pediatric melanoma: risk factor and survival analysis of the surveillance, epidemiology and end results database. J Clin Oncol 2005;23:4735–41.

Su LD, Fullen DR, Sondak VK, Johnson TM, Lowe L. Sentinel lymph node biopsy for patients with problematic spitzoid melanocytic lesions: a report on 18 patients. Cancer 2003;97:499–507.

Swerdlow AJ, English JS, Qiao Z. The risk of melanoma in patients with congenital nevi: a cohort study. J Am Acad Dermatol 1995;32:595–9.

Tannous ZS, Mihm MC, Sober AJ, Duncan LM. Congenital melanocytic nevi: clinical and histopathologic features, risk of melanoma, and clinical management. J Am Acad Dermatol 2005;52:197–203.

Urso C, Borgognoni L, Saieva C, et al. Sentinel lymph node biopsy in patients with 'atypical Spitz tumors'. A report on 12 cases. Hum Pathol 2006;37:816–23.

Vourc'h-Jourdain M, Martin L, Barbarot S. aRED. Large congenital melanocytic nevi: therapeutic management and melanoma risk: a systematic review. J Am Acad Dermatol 2013;68. 493-8.e1-14.

Waelchli R, Aylett SE, Atherton D, Thompson DJ, Chong WK, Kinsler VA. Classification of neurological abnormalities in children with congenital melanocytic naevus syndrome identifies magnetic resonance imaging as the best predictor of clinical outcome. Br J Dermatol 2015;173(3):739–50.

Wiesner T, He J, Yelensky R, et al. Kinase fusions are frequent in Spitz tumors and spitzoid melanomas. Nat Commun 2014;5:3116.

Wong JR, Harris JK, Rodriguez-Galindo C, et al. Incidence of childhood and adolescent melanoma in the United States: 1973–2009. Pediatrics 2013;131:846–54.

Yagerman S, Marghoob AA. Melanoma at the periphery of a congenital melanocytic nevus. J Am Acad Dermatol 2013;69:e227–8.

Yélamos O, Arva NC, Obregon R, et al. A comparative study of proliferative nodules and lethal melanomas in congenital nevi from children. Am J Surg Pathol 2015;39(3):405–15.

Yun SJ, Kwon OS, Han JH, et al. Clinical characteristics and risk of melanoma development from giant congenital melanocytic naevi in Korea: a nationwide retrospective study. Br J Dermatol 2012;166:115–23.

Zaal LH, Mooi WJ, Klip H, van der Horst CM. Risk of malignant transformation of congenital melanocytic nevi: a retrospective nationwide study from The Netherlands. Plast Reconstr Surg 2005;116:1902–9.

7.5

Management of Metastatic Melanoma With Unknown Primary

Luc Thomas, Stephane Dalle

Lyon 1 University, Cancer Research Center of Lyon, Lyon, France

1 NOSOLOGY

Discovery of lymph node or visceral malignant invasion by melanoma cells without clear previous history of cutaneous, ocular, or mucosal melanoma is not an uncommon situation [1]. In such a case the four possible explanations for this phenomenon are the following:

- Neglected or left undiagnosed primary tumor or misdiagnosed primary tumor (Hutchinson's melanotic whitlow)
- Fully or almost fully regressed primary tumor
- Metastatic spread from a visceral (occult) primary tumor (eye, sinuses, gastrointestinal tract, meninges, etc.)
- Hypothetical primary melanoma (them unique) of the lymph node or the affected organ

2 POSITIVE DIAGNOSIS

Careful reevaluation of the possible differential histopathological diagnoses is certainly the most important first step in the management of such cases:

- Clear cell sarcoma of the aponeuroses [2] is a primary tumor of the soft tissues that shares with melanoma cytological as well as immunopathological features.
- Other histopathological differential diagnoses are in most cases solved by immunohistochemistry: melan-A, S-100, and HMB-45; yet undifferentiated lesions might be difficult to identify.

- Genotypic study (bRAF, cKIT, nRAS, etc.) and other therapeutic-linked special tests (PDL-1) could/should be then done.

3 GENERAL RULES OF MANAGEMENT

After clear histopathological confirmation of the diagnosis the initial workout has two goals:

- Identification of a possible primary in patient's history and at patient's examination
- Identification of other visceral or nodal involvement

4 HISTORY

Patient's interrogation should be thorough and search for:

- History of skin surgery for pigmented or unpigmented tumor, and then review of the histopathological slides
- History of destruction of any skin lesion for cosmetical reason(s) without pathology examination (LASER, cryotherapy, etc.)
- History of growing, and then regressed pigmented or unpigmented lesion of the skin [3]
- Recent impairment of vision
- Recent change in the digestive function
- Recent change or trouble in the upper respiratory function
- Any other unusual internal change

5 SKIN EXAMINATION

Since most cases of primary melanoma are cutaneous, clinical examination should include thorough full skin examination with special attention to the skin draining into the involved lymph node basin in case of lymph node tumor.

Skin examination should search for the following:

- An obvious [neglected or hardly visible to patient's eye (Fig. 7.5.1)] primary melanoma
- Presence of a large congenital nevus (the primary melanoma can be within the nevus, in a satellite, or on the meningeal)
- Examination of the oral cavity, perianal and genital skin
- Dermoscopical examination of all pigmented or unpigmented skin lesions

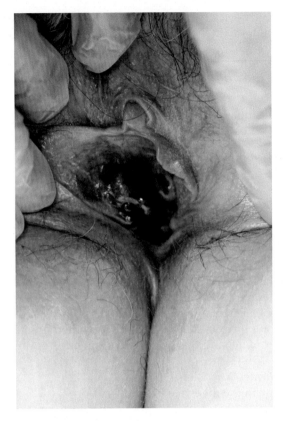

FIGURE 7.5.1   **Primary vulvar advanced melanoma unknown from the patient and her doctors and revealed by liver and adrenal metastases.**

- Surgical or trauma-induced scars with patient's interrogation about the origin of each of them
- Unexplained atrophic or erythematous scar-like lesions with at dermoscopical examination: granulation "peppering", telangiectasias, white shiny streaks "chrysalis" (Fig. 7.5.2) [3]
- Vitiligo (especially atypical vitiligoid depigmentation) (Fig. 7.5.3)
- Skin metastases
- Melanoderma (+black discoloration of urine)

6 SEARCH FOR ANOTHER COMMON EXTRACUTANEOUS PRIMARY

If skin examination is negative, it is often proposed to search for the three most common primary sites after skin (eye, sinuses, genitalia) [4]:

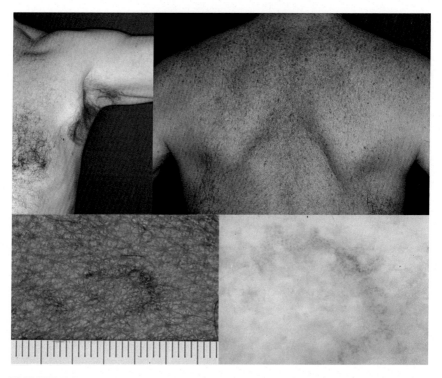

FIGURE 7.5.2 Metastatic melanoma to the left axillary lymph nodes (*upper left*); presence of an unexplained scar on the back (*upper right and lower left image*); dermoscopy shows scar-like depigmentation, pink color of the background, and peppering. Final diagnosis was completely regressed melanoma with lymph node involvement.

- Ophthalmological examination
- Gynecological examination (in males inspection of the genitals does not require specialist examination)
- Endoscopy of the facial sinuses by an otorhinolaryngologist

Since precise identification of the primary does not change the prognosis or the management if the melanoma is not cutaneous, mucosal, or ocular, other explorations (endoscopy, imaging, etc.) will be performed only in case of clinical symptoms. Moreover, whole body PET-CT imaging (see underneath) may help to identify some rare types of primary visceral melanomas (especially gastrointestinal, pleural, or bronchial).

7 INITIAL WORKOUT AND STAGING

Other visceral or nodal involvement should be searched for in the initial workout:

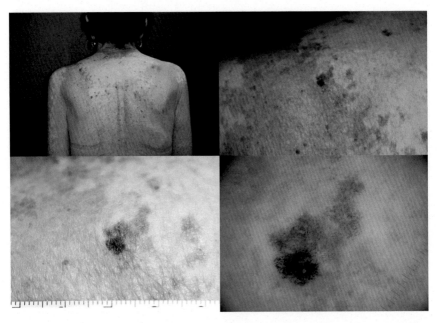

FIGURE 7.5.3   **Patient with recent surgery of a left axillary enlarged lymph node; initial workout also disclosed lung and liver secondary cancer.** Histopathological examination of the lymph node concluded to melanoma. Clinical examination of the skin shows vitiligoid skin depigmentation a classical paraneoplastic syndrome in melanoma and a gray macule of the back (*upper left and right and lower left*). Dermoscopy shows scar-like depigmentation, white shiny streaks ("chrysalis"), and gray granulation ("peppering"). Final diagnosis was almost completely regressive primary melanoma with multifocal metastatic disease.

- Complete clinical examination.
- Any appropriate test (imaging, nuclear medicine, endoscopy, etc.) in case of clinical symptom.
- FDG PET–CT imaging of the whole body is nowadays the key staging test (and can suggest an occult primary site in some cases) [5].
- Chest CT is often added since PET is slightly less efficient for lung examination.
- MRI or CT scan of the brain is systematically added.

General rules of the AJCC-UICC-TNM staging apply ("Tx" in case of definitively unidentified or unidentifiable primary tumor) [6].

8 THERAPEUTIC MANAGEMENT

There is now good evidence that the prognosis of metastatic melanoma with unknown primary is similar and even slightly better to the prognosis of melanoma with known primary [1]; therefore the management will follow the same rules [7,8]:

- Lymph node dissection of the whole involved lymph node basin in case of lymph node involvement, and then discussion in a multidisciplinary tumor board of an eventual inclusion in a clinical trial for adjuvant therapy and follow-up
- If feasible, complete surgical excision of a unique or localized visceral metastasis, and then discussion in a multidisciplinary tumor board of an eventual inclusion in a clinical trial for adjuvant therapy and follow-up
- If unresectable (plurifocal, impossible surgery), discussion, in a multidisciplinary tumor board, of a systemic treatment by immunotherapy or anti-BRAF/MEK targeted therapy (ideally in the setting of a clinical trial) and follow-up

References

[1] Bae JM, Choi YY, Kim DS, Lee JH, Jang HS, Lee JH, et al. Metastatic melanomas of unknown primary show better prognosis than those of known primary: a systematic review and meta-analysis of observational studies. J Am Acad Dermatol 2015;72(1):59–70.
[2] Kosemehmetoglu K, Folpe AL. Clear cell sarcoma of tendons and aponeuroses, and osteoclast-rich tumour of the gastrointestinal tract with features resembling clear cell sarcoma of soft parts: a review and update. J Clin Pathol 2010;63(5):416–23.
[3] Bories N, Dalle S, Debarbieux S, Balme B, Ronger-Savlé S, Thomas L. Dermoscopy of fully regressive cutaneous melanoma. Br J Dermatol 2008;158(6):1224–9.
[4] Kibbi N, Kluger H, Choi JN. Melanoma: clinical presentations. Cancer Treat Res 2016;167:107–29.
[5] Jouvet JC, Thomas L, Thomson V, Yanes M, Journe C, Morelec I, et al. Whole-body MRI with diffusion-weighted sequences compared with 18 FDG PET-CT, CT and superficial lymph node ultrasonography in the staging of advanced cutaneous melanoma: a prospective study. J Eur Acad Dermatol Venereol 2014;28(2):176–85.
[6] Balch CM, Gershenwald JE, Soong SJ, Thompson JF. Update on the melanoma staging system: the importance of sentinel node staging and primary tumor mitotic rate. J Surg Oncol 2011;104(4):379–85.
[7] Harries M, Malvehy J, Lebbe C, Heron L, Amelio J, Szabo Z, et al. Treatment patterns of advanced malignant melanoma (stage III–IV)—a review of current standards in Europe. Eur J Cancer 2016;60:179–89.
[8] Kamposioras K, Pentheroudakis G, Pectasides D, Pavlidis N. Malignant melanoma of unknown primary site. To make the long story short. A systematic review of the literature. Crit Rev Oncol Hematol 2011;78(2):112–26.

Index